Ruminant formula for the future: nutrition or pathology?

Ruminant formula for the future: nutrition or pathology?

Elevating performance and health

edited by:
Sylvie Andrieu
Helen Warren

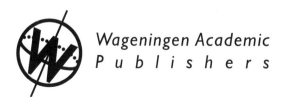

Wageningen Academic
P u b l i s h e r s

ISBN: 978-90-8686-105-7

First published, 2009

© Wageningen Academic Publishers
The Netherlands, 2009

Contents

Improving cattle health: knowledge transfer and motivation

T.J.G.M. Lam[1], J. Jansen[2], J.C.L. Van Veersen[1] and C.D.M. Steuten[2]
[1]Dutch Udder Health Center, P.O. Box 2030, 7420 AA Deventer, the Netherlands
[2]Communication Science, Wageningen University, P.O. Box 8130 6700 EW Wageningen, the Netherlands

1. Introduction

Worldwide, many activities are undertaken to improve cattle health, varying from research projects to knowledge-transfer programs, herd health advisory programs and cow-based ambulatory work. Although much energy is spent on curing diseased animals, the most important part of veterinary medicine is prevention. To stimulate activities in the field of preventive medicine, it is not enough to create knowledge. The knowledge has to be transferred to farmers. This, however, demands a pro-active role of both farmer and advisor, be it a veterinarian or another advisor.

Although the veterinarian is seen as the most important advisor on cattle health by many farmers, their role is mainly reactive (Steuten *et al.*, 2008). If a farmer, for instance, perceives an udder health problem and is motivated to solve that problem, the local practitioner is the first one to be contacted and he or she will try to help the farmer out (Jansen *et al.*, 2004). The level at which udder health is perceived as a problem, however, differs strongly among farmers (Huijps *et al.*, 2008). Many farmers are not convinced of the importance of udder health beyond the visible level, thus it does not lead to action from them. Generally, veterinary practitioners are not the ones to pro-actively show farmers possible gains in this field. Many practitioners think they are unable to convince their clients of the possible (economic) profits from investing in cattle health (Mee, 2007).

In research, much attention is given to further development of veterinary knowledge, while the attention for the transfer of the developed knowledge, although crucial (LeBlanc *et al.*, 2006), is limited. For a number of reasons, motivation and education of farmers have not easy and are challenges on at least two levels. First, farmers who are basically willing to improve animal health still need to be convinced to actually put a lot of energy in prevention programs. Activities, such as conducting an accurate administration of disease cases, scoring teat or body condition on a regular basis, or calculating treatment successes, are not first nature for many farmers. In a study on lameness in 49 herds by Barker *et al.* (2007) for instance, after clinical training only a quarter of all recommendations were implemented, most of which were small, one-time changes or low cost interventions (L. Green, personal communication). Second, to improve cattle health at a national level, as many farmers as possible need to be involved in a program. To reach that goal, farmers not only need to be motivated and educated to carry out herd health programs, but many of them need to be motivated to put the subject on the agenda at all. Knowing how to solve animal health problems, such as mastitis, is generally not the bottle-neck (Green *et al.*, 2007). Knowledge-transfer is.

A specific role is the one of the private practitioner, because of his changing role over the years. In today's veterinary practice, herd health management becomes more and more important. In many parts of the world dairy farmers don't make much money, so practitioners simply become too expensive to do routine work that others can do just as well. A number of traditional veterinary skills move to less expensive workers and, although denied by some, practitioners have no choice but to evolve to advice-oriented consultants (LeBlanc *et al.*, 2006) in order to stay in business. To be successful in that, knowledge from different disciplines must be integrated in recommendations and advice. Successful herd health and production management programs require understanding of each farm as an integrated system (Brand *et al.*, 1996). Additionally, veterinarians need to have the skills to motivate farmers, to transfer knowledge and to sell this advice as a product. A complicating factor is that over the last decades, while veterinarians moved from treatment of clinical illness to disease prevention and from individual cows to herd level, the farmer moved to a more active and independent role. He is by no means any longer obedient to, or impressed by, the veterinarian. This means that the practitioner really has to convince the client of the added value of his or her advice. Of course practitioners try to convince farmers of the importance of the advice given, generally by explaining the veterinary background to it. That is, however, not enough if you want the advice to be executed, and certainly not if you are looking for new clients for advice-consultancy work or new participants in animal health programs. Many practitioners find it difficult to take the step to become more advice-oriented. Quite a few lack 'belief in own capacities', as described by Mee (2007) in relation to providing specialized fertility services. In that same study, practitioners mentioned that when clients did not demand programs, this was a valid reason not to offer them. These practitioners did not consider themselves good 'salesmen'. They probably were right.

This paper will provide some insights and opportunities for different approaches in knowledge transfer and motivation of dairy farmers regarding animal health. We will focus on three issues: (a) the need to adapt the content of communication to farmers' motivation and mindset, (b) different types of communication and the adaptation to the needs of the farmer, and (c) the importance of the source of information and the need to adapt it to the character of the farmer.

2. Farmers' motivation and mindset

Motivation is an important element in changing people's behaviour. Figure 1 shows that behavioural change can be induced by several policy instruments. In this model, behaviour (i.e. the implementation of preventive programs on cattle health) can be influenced via compulsory or voluntary means (Leeuwis, 2004; Van Woerkum *et al.*, 1999). Compulsory behavioural change is facilitated by coercion, such as regulations and restrictive provisions (Van Woerkum *et al.*, 1999). In Bulk Milk Somatic Cells Counts (BMSCC) programs the effect of milk quality legislation and control systems can be more or less subscribed to coercion. However, it is well known that compulsory behavioural change will

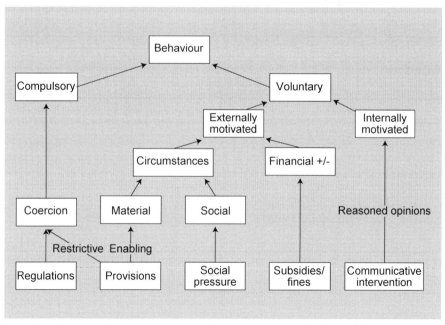

Figure1. Behavioural change by policy instruments (Leeuwis, 2004; Van Woerkum et al., *1999).*

probably only last as long as the coercion exists. Additionally, with respect to udder health, coercion can only be used in extreme cases and only for bulk milk parameters. Thus, voluntary behavioural change is much preferred.

Voluntary behavioural change is induced by either internal and/or external motivation. External motivation can, for instance, be accomplished by financial means through bonuses and penalties related to BMSCC (Schukken *et al.*, 1992). When asked, farmers are convinced that if they received premiums for lower cell counts, they would be motivated to react (Jansen *et al.*, 2004). A study of Valeeva *et al.* (2007), however, showed that quality penalties tended to be more effective in motivating farmers to change their behaviour than quality premiums.

Internal motivation can be influenced by communicative intervention through reasoned opinions, such as persuading farmers by use of articles in magazines, lectures at informative meetings and in study groups, and discussions with the practitioner. Internal motivation is probably most effective in long-term behavioural change. However, to understand internal motivation of a farmer, we need to understand and anticipate the farmers' 'mindset' and the interaction of farmers with their social environment.

Leeuwis *et al.* (2006) developed a model about decision making of people based on a mindset in interaction with others (see Figure 2). This shows that what people do, or not do, depends on different factors, which are influenced by identity. The model shows that farmers make different decisions based on the identity they have at that moment. For example, a farmer would make a different decision in his role as a father, than in his role as a farmer. This role or identity of a farmer and the accompanying factors are constructed in interaction with the farmer's environment and can, therefore, also be influenced by communication strategies.

Analysis of factors influencing the mindset of farmers in relation to the Dutch udder health program learned that the Leeuwis model could be applied. For 'risk perception' a difference is found between the problem-level and the satisfaction level, for instance for BMSCC the levels are on average 280,000 and 150,000 cells/ml, respectively (Jansen *et al.*, 2004). We found that only 27% of farmers managed to reach their satisfactory level, while 6% of the farmers violate their problem level. The way farmers perceive risks plays a crucial role in this as risk assessments are situationally sensitive expressions of personal value systems. Optimistic bias (it won't happen to me), as well as a lack of 'trust in

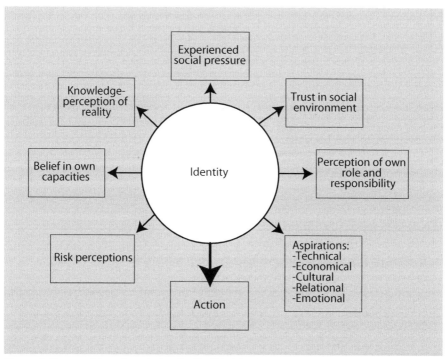

Figure 2. Composition of a mindset by flexible identities in interaction processes (Leeuwis et al., 2006).

the social environment', such as institutions and experts can be an obstacle in effective communication (Hansen *et al.*, 2003).

Evaluation of 'belief in own capacities' in a questionnaire on udder health showed that 27% of the dairy farmers think they directly know what the causes are when a mastitis problem occurs and 32% of the farmers in the survey think they know enough about mastitis to prevent problems (Jansen *et al.*, 2004). These results suggest that about two-thirds of Dutch dairy farmers feel insecure about actually dealing with mastitis management. This corresponds with the findings on 'knowledge perception of reality'. Most farmers think they have sufficient knowledge about mastitis in general but that this knowledge is not always decisive in relation to their own situation (Jansen *et al.*, 2004).

The positive results found in study-groups of farmers (Lam *et al.*, 2007) reinforce the fundaments of communication theories that 'experienced social pressure' by colleagues and social learning are important in persuasion. Additional factors explaining farmers' behaviour are 'perception of own role and responsibility' and 'aspirations'. Results from the baseline survey showed that most important farm objectives are to get a high net return and to keep the farm management simple (Jansen *et al.*, 2004). This can be conflicting with the messages in cattle health programs. Farmers may perceive the application of extra preventive measures to be expensive or complicated. Realising that farmers are as diverse as other people and that that not all farmers are motivated to 'understand' would be a big step forward.

Based on the above, a farmer's mindset can then be seen as a combination of what farmers want, know, believe and perceive regarding cattle health. As such, the mindset can support the understanding of farmers' behaviour and the way this behaviour can be influenced.

3. Different types of communication adapted to farmers' needs

To motivate people to work on mastitis, it is important that you know how to communicate your message. Everyone, including farmers, has a preferred way to obtain information. Some might prefer abstract information, like numbers and figures, while others want to see the real thing, e.g. 'how does my herd look today'. These different ways to obtain information can be described as learning styles (Kolb, 1984). Communication with farmers should be adapted to these learning styles. In our opinion many advisors, especially veterinary practitioners ask too few questions to be able to differentiate between farmers (Steuten *et al.*, 2008). It is then hard to choose the best approach without knowing what the farmer wants and what his preferred learning style is. This is assuming an approach is actually chosen. To convince farmers of the value of the advice given, veterinary practitioners tend not to choose and to follow one strategy: explaining the technical background of the matter. Too often it is assumed that, once the farmer understands, he or she will act likewise. The background of this is comparable to the expert-lay discrepancy as described for food risks (Hansen *et al.*, 2003). The expert-lay discrepancy is often attributed to a 'knowledge deficit' among 'lay people' (farmers). Reality is much more complex.

Motivation to work on cattle health can be influenced to a certain level (see above). Given (and taking into account) the level of motivation, one tries to reach farmers as well as possible. Therefore, an important factor in knowledge transfer is the way people learn most easily and thus the way knowledge is presented. Kolb (1984) differentiates four learning styles: accommodator, diverger, converger, and assimilator (Figure 3), which will be discussed below. The Kolb theory holds that an individual's ability to learn will be enhanced by strategies that conform to the individual's preferred learning style.

An accommodator is very practically orientated, he or she learns by experience. He is the type of person who tries to get a machine running before reading the manual, 'trial and error' is preferred. Offering the possibility to experiment actively and to have concrete experiences is a way to reach the accommodator (Van Helden, 1986). Specimens of products you want to be used, like for instance milking gloves or a milk-progesterone test, may be picked up by him.

A diverger learns by weighing up different perspectives. A diverger is accessible via concrete experiences and reflects and analyses these. He likes to approach a problem from different angles and enjoys an environment that asks for creativity. A diverger appreciates analyses of problems in cooperation with others, discussions about different approaches etc. Excursions to model farms or open door days as used by Reneau (2007) in Minnesota can be good learning

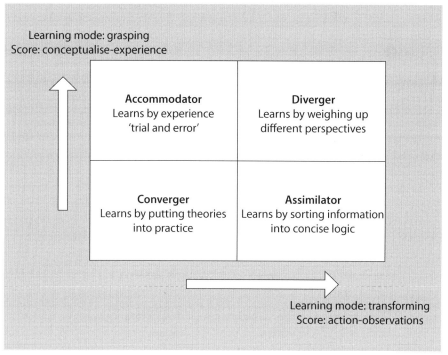

Figure 3. The learning styles according to Kolb (adapted from Paine, 1993 as reference).

methods for him. All persons and organizations in the social environment, including organizations for agricultural and veterinary education, should express the same message. In that way conflicting information is avoided and farmers' trust and motivation in the social environment will be better maintained.

A converger learns by putting theories into practice. He will start reading the manual and will follow it step-by-step. In study-groups on udder health we organized in the Netherlands our experience was that farmers appreciated instructions on basic areas of routine work in animal health (Meesters *et al.*, 2007). Actions the practitioner would initially take for granted like 'where to inject a cow' and 'how to do a CMT' were found very useful, especially if applied using the cows in the barn. This can be interpreted as a mixture of a converging and a diverging learning style. Tools specific for convergers can be instruction cards or treatment schedules. Van Helden (1986) describes that thinking in concepts and generalisations are important for convergers. In learning they prefer questions with only one correct answer. Practical implications of the content are very important for them.

Finally, an assimilator learns by sorting information into concise logic. The assimilator is the more scientific type. He or she appreciates observation and reflection to form conceptual ideas. Assimilators want to gather lots of information from different sources, they like self-study, and will gradually form an idea on the subject (Van Helden, 1986). An advisor is only one source of information. He will use more than one advisor and other sources of information. The internet, with websites with technical information, articles in farmers' magazines, information at dairy shows, agricultural education, information given by the dairy industry and farmers organizations will all be absorbed and weighted.

One would expect most farmers to be accommodators (Paine, 1993). However, a study on learning styles of sheep and beef cattle farmers in New Zealand showed that of 81 participants of study groups a surprising 50% expressed a preference for logical learning (assimilator) (Webby and Paine, 1997). It would be easier in knowledge transfer if all people were alike, a wish that is often translated into practice. In trying to be successful in knowledge transfer and in changing the behaviour of different types of farmers, however, one needs to take all learning styles into account.

4. The source of information

Farmers gather knowledge from different sources, among which their veterinary practitioner plays an important role (Jansen *et al.*, 2004). Communication and understanding between farmer and advisor is essential (Vaarst *et al.*, 2002). Even when an advisor takes the farmers' motivation into account, and participates optimally on different learning styles, a 'hard to reach' group will remain. Trying to find out more about this phenomena, a group of farmers, considered as hard to reach by veterinary practitioners, was interviewed. The farmers' opinion and attitude towards udder health, the role of the veterinary practitioner and other advisors, the way they use sources of information and how they are influenced by their social environment was studied. These 'hard to reach' farmers were classified based on their orientation towards the outside world and their trust in external information sources into four categories: do-it-yourselfer, information seeker, wait-and-see-er, or individualist (see Figure 4). The attitude and approach of the farmers in the different groups towards their veterinarian is described below. Additionally some thoughts on how to approach the different groups are given.

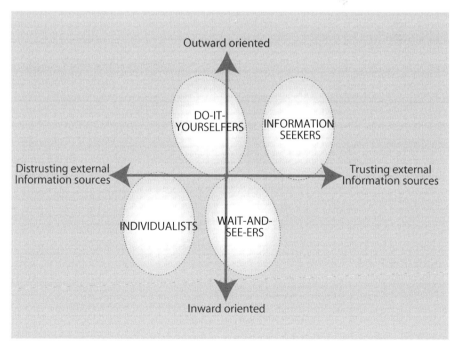

Figure 4. Categories of farmers who are perceived as 'hard to reach', by veterinary practitioners.

The do-it-yourselfer does not specifically have anything against the veterinary practitioner and will not hesitate to ask advice of his veterinarian when he perceives the benefits higher than the costs. He tends, however, to rely more on his own experience and knowledge than to accept advice from others in general. Only some of them feel that they have a relationship of trust with their veterinarian. They perceive high costs of the veterinarian as an important argument to call the veterinarian as little as possible to their farm. The same is probably true for other advisors. To reach this group, a businesslike approach is most suitable. That is the way they act themselves and appreciate to be approached. To raise their attention locally organized field demonstrations or 'open door days' are probably a good approach.

Information seekers are well informed and interested in new developments in different fields. They are interested in the opinion of others and do not object to the veterinarian or others knowing the details of their farm administration. Generally, they consider the relation with their veterinarian as informative and good. However, other advisors, study groups and colleagues are also considered as important sources of information on cattle health. Most farmers in this group make use of the internet as an information source. The reason they are considered as hard to reach by their veterinarian may be the fact they also use many information sources other than their veterinarian. To reach this group one should realize there are different advisors in the field of cattle health, and try to look for cooperation. Making information available from various sources, which are easy accessible is the best way to change behaviour in this group.

Individualists try to keep the veterinarian off their farm as much as possible, as they do with every other 'external person'. They try to give other people as little access to their farm information as possible. These farmers do not feel that they have a relationship of trust with their veterinarian or any other advisor. As such, intensive interpersonal communication with these farmers might be less effective. It is remarkable, however, that these farmers, as most others, are interested in what happens in the outside world. They read agricultural journals, especially articles that describe other farms. Subsequently, the best way to reach these farmers is through farm magazines and not by interpersonal communication.

The wait-and-see-er is basically interested and feels he ought to do more with animal health but he finds it hard to put advice into practice, especially in the long term. He lacks internal motivation, thus he needs extra stimulation from outside to come to action. The often heard approach among veterinary practitioners that 'farmers know what services we offer and they either call us to deliver those services, or they don't' certainly won't work here. Intensive personal communication, as well as social pressure through the presentation of successful examples on other farms may help to bring this group to action.

Interesting to note is that all 'hard to reach' farmers read agricultural journals. These are mentioned as the most important information source for all farmers in this group. However, besides using these journals, the different groups need to be approached differently. The results of this study show that for these 'hard to reach' farmers, the veterinary practitioner may not have realized the importance of motivation and mindset, like in the group of information seekers and wait-and-seers. For them, a proactive approach would probably have been more successful than a reactive one. Also, learning styles may not have been fully elaborated. It may, for instance, be successful to approach the group of do-it-yourselfers as being accommodators. Finally, the veterinary practitioner was not the right source of information for a number of the farmers in this specific group. Some veterinarians don't take the effort or are unable to handle the difficult communication issues described above. We found striking differences between different veterinary practices in activities, showing that if veterinarians seize the opportunity, by investing in a customer oriented commercial approach, they will increase their credibility and their client satisfaction. Although not evaluated in the study described above, the same probably is true for other advisors.

5. Discussion

To improve cattle health at the population level, it is important to understand farmers. It is not only important to know what motivates them, it is also important to know how farmers like to learn and which information sources they use. To reach that goal, all advisors in the farmer's social network are important. These are veterinarians, nutritionists, artificial insemination technicians, salesmen, cattle traders, milking machine advisors and so on. We experienced that farmers are influenced by many different people (including advisors), and that they differ in susceptibility to the influence of these people. To actually improve cattle health it is important that all these people send the same message, which is customized to the farmers needs. On many occasions, however, it is difficult to find consensus among advisors.

Although advisors often are very aware of the differences between farmers in the way they ought to be motivated to adopt disease prevention programs, they often seem to be unable to adapt their advisory strategy to the different farmer types. Some farmers give top priority to animal health and related programs, and have a proactive and enthusiastic relationship with their advisor. Others only contact their advisor when serious problems occur, being it animal health or other issues (prize, product quality, etc.).

In animal health advising by veterinary practitioners or others, communication plays an important role. Generally the advisors do have the knowledge available and have access to the farmers. Practitioners have shown to be able to improve udder health results of internally motivated farmers (Green *et al.*, 2007; Lam *et al.*, 2007). Veterinary practitioners themselves find it difficult to motivate farmers who are not interested in the first place. There may be possibilities to intensify the contact with that group of farmers (Mee, 2007). As described above, if communication is not successful it may be the result of the farmer, like for instance in the case of 'individualists' who appear not to trust anybody. On the other hand, there also seem to be farmers that are basically willing to participate in all kind of activities, but have not been approached in the optimal way. The available knowledge in the field of motivation, mindset and learning styles has not been applied. In a changing agricultural world, the need for effective knowledge transfer and motivation of farmers increases. Currently, many cattle health programs focus on expert-to-lay communication, including the perception that farmers have limited knowledge and that they will adopt the provided knowledge instantly once they understand the background. This misconception leads to communication programs which are one-sided and only attracts farmers with the accompanying learning style.

Motivation and behaviour varies between farmers, is quite unpredictable, context related and not easy to influence in a short period of time. As such, it should be acknowledged that it is inevitable that we need to use a combination of communication strategies to change farmers' behaviour. Additionally, one has to anticipate the farmers' mindset regarding animal health. Changing people's behaviour by improving motivation and knowledge transfer is not impossible, as long as we recognize the differences between famers and take that into account as individual advisors. This demands a pro-active role of advisors, but also needs changes in current and future communication programs to improve cattle health. All these factors have to be taken in to account when trying to improve cattle health, but are also important for the individual advisors with his or her own specific role.

Acknowledgements

This report is part of the five year mastitis program of the Dutch Udder Health Centre and was financially supported by the Dutch Dairy Board.

References

Barker, Z.E., J.R. Amory, J.L. Wright, R.W Blowey and L.E. Green, 2007. Management factors associated with impaired locomotion in dairy cows in England and Wales. *Journal of Dairy Science* **90**:3270-3277.

Brand, A., J.P.T.M. Noordhuizen and Y.H. Schukken, 1996. Herd Health and Production Management in Dairy Practice. Wageningen Pers, the Netherlands.

Green, M.J., K.A. Leach, J.E. Breen, L.E. Green, and A.J. Bradley, 2007. National intervention study of mastitis control in dairy herds in England and Wales. *Veterinary Record* **160**:287-93.

Hansen, J., L. Holm, L. Frewer, P. Robinson and P. Sandøe, 2003. Beyond the knowledge deficit: recent research into lay and expert attitudes to food risks. *Appetite* **41**:111-121.

Huijps, K., T.J.G.M. Lam. and H. Hogeveen, 2008. Costs of mastitis: facts and perception. *Journal of Dairy Research* **75**:113-120.

Jansen, J., Kuiper, D., Renes, R.J. and Leeuwis,C., 2004. Report baseline survey mastitis: knowledge, attitude, behaviour (in Dutch). Wageningen University, the Netherlands.

Kolb, D., 1984. Experimental learning. Prentice-Hall., New Jersey.

Lam, T.J.G.M., J. Jansen, B.H.P. Van den Borne and J.H.L. Van Veersen, 2007. A structural approach of udder health improvement via private practitioners: ups and downs. Proceedings NMC, January 21-24, San Antonio, Texas, USA. pp. 142- 151.

LeBlanc, S.J., K.D. Lissemore, D.F. Kelton, T.F. Duffield and K.E. Leslie, 2006. Major advances in disease prevention in dairy cattle. *Journal of Dairy Science* **89**:1267-1279.

Leeuwis, C., 2004. Communication for rural innovation. Rethinking agricultural extension. Oxford, Blackwell Science Ltd.

Leeuwis, C., R. Smits, J. Grin, L. Klerkx, B. Van Mierlo, and A. Kuipers, 2006. Equivocations on the post privatization dynamics in agricultural innovation systems. Transforum Working Papers, Zoetermeer, the Netherlands.

Mee, J.F., 2007. The role of the veterinarian in bovine fertility management on modern dairy farms. *Theriogenology* **68**(S1):257-265.

Meesters, A.J.M., J. Jansen, J. Van Veersen and T.J.G.M. Lam, 2007. How to organize successful study-group meetings with dairy farmers: experiences on udder health. Proceedings Cattle Consultancy Days, Aarhus, Denmark.

Paine, M.S., 1993. Extension agents can perform more effectively through an appreciation of individual learning styles. Proceedings New Zealand Society of Animal Production. pp. 115-119.

Reneau, J.K., 2007. Quality Count$: a SCC reducing campaign in Minnesota. Proceedings NMC, January 21-24, San Antonio, Texas, USA, pp. 136-141.

Schukken, Y.H., K.E. Leslie, A.J. Weersink, and S.W. Martin, 1992. Ontario bulk milk somatic cell count reduction program. I. Impact on somatic cell counts and milk quality. *Journal of Dairy Science* 75:3352-3358.

Steuten, C.D.M., J. Jansen, R.J. Renes, M.N.C. Aarts and T.J.G.M. Lam, 2008. Effective communication with 'hard-to-reach' farmers. In: *Mastitis control*, T.J.G.M. Lam (ed.), Wageningen Academic Publishers, Wageningen, the Netherlands, pp. 389-395.

Vaarst, M., B. Paarup-Laursen, H. Houe, C. Fossing and H.J. Andersen, 2002. Farmers' choice of medical treatment of mastitis in Danish dairy herds based on qualitative research interviews. *Journal of Dairy Science* 85:992-1001.

Valeeva, N.I., H. Hogeveen and T.J.G.M. Lam, 2007. Motivation of Dairy Farmers to Improve Mastitis Management. *Journal of Dairy Science* 90:4466-4477.

Van Helden, H.J., 1986. Starting mastership – differentiation of learning styles (in Dutch). Free University of Amsterdam, the Netherlands.

Van Woerkum, C., D. Kuiper and E. Bos, 1999. Communication and innovation: an introduction (in Dutch). Samsom, Alphen aan de Rijn, the Netherlands.

Webby, R.W. and M.S. Paine, 1997. Farmer groups: a measure of their effectiveness. Proceedings New Zealand Society of Animal Production. pp. 109-111.

Managing calf health through nutrition

A.J. Heinrichs
The Pennsylvania State University, Department of Dairy and Animal Science,
0324 Henning Building, University Park, Pennsylvania, USA

1. Introduction

Calf health, as reflected in morbidity and mortality, is a consistent and major issue facing dairy farmers around the world. Data from Europe and the USA clearly show that dairy calf mortality remains above 5-8% year on year representing a significant economic impact on the dairy farm economy (Fourichon *et al.*, 1997; National Animal Health Monitoring System, 2007; Svensson *et al.*, 2006) and, in addition, morbidity remains high, which adds to the economic burden through added labour and health supply costs; and over 50% of this morbidity is related to neonatal scours (Losinger and Heinrichs, 1996). Nutrition of the dry cow and newborn calf can have direct influences on the morbidity and mortality of the calf.

2. Colostrum

When calf health is discussed, we must begin with the nutrition of the dam and the related influence on the body tissues of the calf at birth and the nutrient value of colostrum. Research has shown that various aspects related to dry cow nutrition can affect the tissue nutrient stores of the calf at birth. Of the various nutrients in calf tissue stores and colostrum, the ones that can be most affected by dry cow diet are the minerals. Protein, lactose and fat levels are difficult to influence in colostrum as a result of diet, however, other aspects of colostrum composition can be modified including vitamins and minerals (Kehoe and Heinrichs, 2007).

Most minerals are water-soluble and, therefore, easily pass through the placental membrane. The foetus is able to store minerals *in utero* and is most often born with sufficient stores. In areas with dietary deficiencies of certain minerals, neonates can easily have problems with these mineral deficiencies. Mineral content in general is high in colostrum and the concentration of most minerals decrease shortly after the onset of lactation to concentrations found in mature bovine milk. Calcium, phosphorus, copper and iron are all generally high with concentrations at 0.16 g/dl, 0.17 g/dl, 0.39 µg/ml and 1.9 µg/ml, respectively, but drop to levels found in mature milk within 25 hours (Foley and Otterby, 1978). Conversely, manganese is one mineral, which has been reported at 0.09 µg/ml (Kincaid and Cronrath, 1992), is not found in higher concentrations in colostrum than in mature milk.

Selenium and iodine are two minerals that can vary widely according to geographic location and the geochemical environment. Much research has reported effects of supplementing gestating farm animals with selenium and the increase of selenium in colostrum (Mahan, 2000; Weiss and Hogan, 2005). Austin *et al.* (1980) reported that supplementing cows with iodine increased colostrum concentrations of iodine; however, calves received most of the iodine found in plasma from placental transfer *in utero* rather than colostrum ingestion. Health issues related to white muscle disease that were once common problems in newborn calves in Se deficient areas are rarely a problem now due to dietary Se supplementation of the dry cow.

Concentrations of fat-soluble vitamins are highly variable between individuals and are also dependent on maternal reserve status, diet and season. Stewart and McCallum (1938) reported variations of retinol from 35 to 1,181 IU/100 ml of colostrum between individual cows on the same management system; this highlights inter-sample variation of fat-soluble vitamins. Weiss *et al.* (1992) also found a significant correlation between fat in colostrum and fat-soluble vitamin concentrations. Due to the close connection of fat-soluble vitamin absorption with the presence of fat in the diet, fat needs to be accounted for when analyzing fat-soluble vitamin concentrations in colostrum and other fluids. Concentrations of alpha-tocopherol in colostrum reported for cows fed without supplemental alpha-tocopherol and cows fed 1000 IU alpha-tocopherol were 95.6 and 125.4 µg/g fat, respectively. Colostrum concentrations of beta-carotene from these same cows were 49.6 and 23.6 µg/g fat, although the reason for the increase in beta-carotene concentrations in unsupplemented animals is unknown (Weiss *et al.*, 1992). The concentration of vitamin A found in colostrum is related to dietary concentrations of vitamin A, which impacts the concentration of vitamin A in the blood of cows before parturition. Plasma vitamin A in newborn calves is four-fold greater when dams are supplemented with vitamin A prepartum and two-fold greater when supplemented with carotene in the prepartum diet compared to unsupplemented cows (Spielman *et al.*, 1947). Although ruminant placental structure is non-invasive and fat-soluble vitamins are large molecular weight substances, there must be some transport of vitamin A because cows supplemented with dietary vitamin A birth calves with higher plasma and liver stores of vitamin A than unsupplemented cows.

Water-soluble vitamins have not been extensively analyzed in colostrum. Previous to high performance liquid chromatography (HPLC), researchers attempting analysis of water-soluble vitamins used methods, such as rat growth, microbiologic assays, chemical and fluorometric assays. There is also variability in concentrations of water-soluble vitamins due to diet, season and individual animals (Kehoe and Heinrichs, 2007).

Colostrum not only provides passive immunity for the newborn calf, but it can also have profound effects on the development of the neonatal intestine, since it contains a number of bioactive and growth-promoting substances, such as peptide hormones, growth factors, cytokines, steroid hormones, thyroxine, polyamines, enzymes, lactoferrin, lysozymes, insulin, cytokines, IGF-1, IGF-2, oligosaccharides and nuceotides (Koldovsky, 1989; Hagiwara *et al.*, 2000).

Nucleotides are part of the non-protein nitrogen fraction of colostrum and consist of a purine or pyrimidine base, a pentose ring and one to three phosphate groups. Nucleotides are found in high levels in colostrum compared with mature milk. Colostrum has high levels of pyrimidine derivatives, such as UDP-glucose, UDP-galactose and uracil monophosphate (UMP) but low levels of guanosine derivatives, adenosine monophosphate (AMP) and cytosine monophosphate (CMP) (Gil and Uauy, 1995). Levels of UMP and guanosine monophosphate (GMP) decrease as colostrum transitions to milk while orotate monophosphate (OMP) increases to higher levels in mature milk than are found in colostrum. Nucleotides are needed in higher amounts in growing or diseased animals and are found in some feedstuffs. Supplementing nucleotides to newborn calves has been shown to improve function of the gut by allowing for more gut wall tissue growth and improving the ability of the calf to transport more nucleotides across the small intestine walls (Kehoe *et al.*, 2008).

3. Colostrum management

An important calf health issue is colostrum management. There are many clear research publications showing the significant effects of timing, quality and quantity of colostrum fed and its impacts on morbidity, mortality, growth, age at calving and culling of dairy heifers. The cornerstone of a successful colostrum management programme are age of calf at first feeding, volume of colostrum administered and immunoglobulin concentration of the colostrum ingested (Stott *et al.*, 1979a,b,c,d).

Failure of passive transfer (FPT) of colostrum maternal immunoglobulins, resulting from a lack of IgG transfer, occurs in a high percentage of calves due to the way colostrum feeding is managed on dairy farms. The correlation with mortality is very strong and this, along with morbidity, represents a serious economic loss to dairy farmers. Recent studies show that colostrum as fed on dairy farms often is not adequate in immunoglobulin and nutrient levels; and is often high in bacteria, all of which need to be improved with management on the farm (Kehoe *et al.*, 2007). Methods to increase immunoglobulin levels in colostrum are limited due to the genetics of the cow (dam) and physiological conditions of the cow at calving time.

Increased neonatal mortality and morbidity is a well-accepted consequence of failure of passive transfer. Besser and Gay (1994) showed that low post-colostral serum IgG level is a significant risk factor for the development of pneumonia in heifer calves. A study by Wells *et al.* (1996) concluded that lack of colostral feeding was highly associated with neonatal death loss in the United States. Donovan *et al.* (1998), in a prospective study to determine calf-level factors that affected calf health status between birth and 6 months of age, showed that there was a clear association between serum total protein (a measure of colostral immunoglobulin absorption) and mortality. Calves with low serum total protein values (< 50 g/l) were 3 to 6 times more likely to die within the first 6 months of life than those with serum total protein concentrations of >60 g/l. In a study by Nocek *et al.* (1984), calves deprived of colostrum gained body weight (BW) poorly and suffered severe and long episodes of scours and high mortality. Calves fed colostrum with high immunoglobulin gained BW from birth to day 4 while those fed colostrum with low immunoglobulin levels lost BW. Overall severity and duration of scours were less for calves fed colostrum with high compared to low immunoglobulin levels. In another study, Besser and Gay (1985) demonstrated that calves with high serum IgG concentrations had lower mortality rates from both enteritis and respiratory disease than calves with serum concentrations of less than 10 g/l.

4. Liquid and dry calf nutrition

Calf nutrition related to basic feeding also can be addressed in relation to health. Levels of nutrients and types of feeding systems impact health. Both low and high levels of milk/milk replacer feeding have been shown to impact calf health and growth. Feeding with less than 10% of BW per day of liquid feed will result in low rates of BW gain and in situations with added stress, may predispose calves to increased morbidity. Altering diet nutrient levels have not been shown to affect immunity unless the nutrient levels are extremely low or high. Calves fed very high levels of milk replacer have been shown to have a depressed immune function (Foote *et al.*, 2007). Therefore, a moderate level liquid calf feeding is often recommended.

Stimulating dry feed intake, primarily starch-containing grains, will stimulate rumen development in the dairy calf. The transition from a primary monogastric to a ruminant diet has great effects on calf health. Once the dairy calf is weaned, digestive upsets and diarrhoea are minimized due to the function of the rumen and its bacterial population. Grain type and level of feeding will affect rumen development (Lesmeister *et al.*, 2004).

5. Conclusion

Nutrition has a great many effects on the health of the calf and improvements must be considered to reduce the high incidence of morbidity and mortality as found on dairy farms around the world. Colostrum and the management of colostrum feeding are the primary ways that early nutrition of the calf can have a profound effect on the health of the calf. Moderate levels of liquid feeds and rapid rumen development complete the calf health and nutrition relationships that are beneficial to the young dairy calf.

References

Austin, A.R., D.C. Whitehead, Y.L. Le Du and J. Brownlie, 1980. The influence of dietary iodine on iodine in the blood serum of cows and calves in the perinatal period. *Research in Veterinary Science* **28**:128-130.

Besser, T.E. and C.C. Gay, 1985. Septicemic colibacillosis and failure of passive transfer of colostral immunoglobulin in calves. *Veterinary Clinics of North America: Food Animal Practice* **1**(3):445-459.

Besser, T.E. and C.C. Gay, 1994. The importance of colostrum to the health of the neonatal calf. *Veterinary Clinics of North America: Food Animal Practice* **10**(1):107-117.

Donovan, G.A., Dahoo, I.R., Montgomery, D.M. and F.L. Bennett, 1998. Associations between passive immunity and morbidity and mortality in dairy heifers in Florida, USA. *Preventative Veterinary Medicine* **34**:31-46.

Foley, J.A. and D.E. Otterby, 1978. Availability, storage, treatment, composition, and feeding value of surplus colostrum: A review. *Journal of Dairy Science* **61**:1033-1060.

Foote, M.R., B.J. Nonnecke, D.C. Beitz and W.R. Waters, 2007. High growth rate fails to enhance adaptive immune responses of neonatal calves and is associated with reduced lymphocyte viability. *Journal of Dairy Science* **90**:404-417.

Fourichon, C., H. Seegers, F. Beaudeau and N. Bareille, 1997. Newborn calf management, morbidity and mortality in French dairy herds. *Épidémiologie et Santé Animale* **31-32**:05.08.1-3.

Gil, A. and R. Uauy, 1995. Nucleotides and related compounds in human and bovine milks. In: *Handbook of milk composition.* R.G. Jensen (ed.) Academic Press, San Diego, pp. 436-494.

Hagiwara, K., S. Kataoka, H. Yamanaka, R. Kirisawa and H. Iwai, 2000. Detection of cytokines in bovine colostrum. *Veterinary Immunology and Immunopathology* **76**:183-190.

Kehoe, S.I. and A.J. Heinrichs, 2007. Bovine colostrum nutrient composition. *CAB Reviews: Perspectives in Agriculture, Veterinary Science, Nutrition and Natural Resources* **2**: No. 029:1-10.

Kehoe, S.I., B.M. Jayarao and A.J. Heinrichs, 2007. A survey of bovine colostrum composition and colostrum management on Pennsylvania dairy farms. *Journal of Dairy Science* **90**:4108-4116.

Kehoe, S.I., A.J. Heinrichs, C.R. Baunrucker and D.L. Gregor. 2008. Effects of nucleotide supplementation in milk replacers on small intestinal absorptive capacity in dairy calves. *Journal of Dairy Science* **91**:2759-2770.

Kincaid, R.L. and J.D. Cronrath, 1992. Zinc concentration and distribution in mammary secretions of peripartum cows. *Journal of Dairy Science* 75(2):481-484.

Koldovsky, O. 1989. Search for role of milk-borne biologically active peptides for the suckling. *Journal of Nutrition* **119**:1543-1551.

Lesmeister, K.E., A.J. Heinrichs and M.T. Gabler, 2004. Effects of supplemental yeast (*Saccharomyces cerevisiae*) culture on rumen development, growth characteristics, and blood parameters in neonatal dairy calves. *Journal of Dairy Science* **87**:1832-1839.

Losinger, W.C. and A.J. Heinrichs, 1996. The management practices associated with herd milk production as determined from the National Dairy Heifer Evaluation Project. *Journal of Dairy Science* **79**:506-514.

Mahan, D.C., 2000. Effect of organic and inorganic selenium sources and levels on sow colostrum and milk selenium content. *Journal of Animal Science* 78(1):100-105.

National Animal Health Monitoring System, 2007. Dairy 2007. Part 1. Reference of dairy health and management in the United States. USDA:APHIS Veterinary Services, Ft. Collins, CO, USA.

Nocek, J.E., D.G. Braund and R.G. Warner, 1984. Influence of neonatal colostrum administration, immunoglobulin, and continued feeding of colostrum on calf gain, health, and serum protein. *Journal of Dairy Science* **67**:319-333.

Spielman, A.A., J.W. Thomas, J.K. Loosli, F. Whiting, C.L. Norton and K.L. Turk, 1947. The relationship of the prepartum diet to the carotene and vitamin A content of bovine colostrum. *Journal of Dairy Science* **30**:343-350.

Stewart, J., and J. W. McCallum. 1938. The vitamin A content of the colostrum of dairy cows. *Journal of Agricultural Science* **28**:428-436.

Stott, G.H., D.B. Marx, B.E. Menefee and G.T. Nightengale, 1979a. Colostral immunoglobulin transfer in calves I. Period of absorption. *Journal of Dairy Science* **62**:1632-1638.

Stott, G.H., D.B. Marx, B.E. Menefee and G.T. Nightengale, 1979b. Colostral immunoglobulin transfer in calves I. Period of absorption. *Journal of Dairy Science* **62**:1632-1638.

Stott, G.H., D.B. Marx, B.E. Menefee and G.T. Nightengale, 1979c. Colostral immunoglobulin transfer in calves II. The rate of absorption. *Journal of Dairy Science* **62**:1766-1773.

Stott, G.H., D.B. Marx, B.E. Menefee and G.T. Nightengale, 1979d. Colostral immunoglobulin transfer in calves III. Amount of absorption. *Journal of Dairy Science* **62**:1902-1907.

Svensson, C., A. Linder and S.-O. Olsson, 2006. Mortality in Swedish dairy calves and replacement heifers. *Journal of Dairy Science* **89**:4769-4777.

Weiss, W.P. and J.S. Hogan, 2005. Effect of selenium source on selenium status, neutrophil function, and response to intramammary endotoxin challenge of dairy cows. *Journal of Dairy Science* **88**(12):4366-4374.

Weiss, W.P., J.S. Hogan, K.L. Smith, D.A. Todhunter and S.N. Williams, 1992. Effect of supplementing periparturient cows with vitamin E on distribution of alpha-tocopherol in blood. *Journal of Dairy Science* **75**:3479-3485.

Wells, S.J., D.A. Dargatz and S.L. Ott, 1996. Factors associated with mortality to 21 days of life in dairy heifers in the United States. *Preventive Veterinary Medicine* **29**:9-19.

The influence of periparturient nutrition on early lactation pathologies of the dairy cow

F.J. Mulligan, R. Alibrahim and L. O'Grady
Unit of Herd and Veterinary Public Health, School of Agriculture, Food Science and Veterinary Medicine, University College Dublin, Ireland

1. Introduction

The modern high producing dairy cow frequently suffers from ill-health in the periparturient period as a consequence of her tremendous ability to produce milk, the management regimes imposed upon her and the myriad of infectious diseases that she is exposed to at that time. Because many disease events in dairy cattle result in cascade-like sequences, which alter many biological systems within the body, maximum or efficient production is only possible from healthy dairy cattle. As a consequence, whether the driver is better dairy cow welfare, better producer profitability or increased food safety; improved dairy cow health is an absolute necessity. The nutrition and management of dairy cows in the periparturient period has an enormous capacity to alter health status, fertility and productivity. It is this capacity for dairy cow nutrition to prevent disease that makes it a key determinant of producer profitability and dairy cow welfare.

1.1. The periparturient period: a time of great change

The period from three weeks pre- to three weeks post-calving has been defined as the transition period for dairy cows (Grummer, 1995). The importance of this period has been recognised in several review articles (Grummer, 1995; Drackley, 1999; Ingvartsen *et al.*, 2003). It is within this period that most disease conditions of dairy cows become evident. This has been documented by Ingvartsen *et al.* (2003) who summarised data from 93,000 first parity and 58,000 third parity Danish dairy cows that demonstrated the highest incidence of total disease (mastitis, ketosis, digestive disorders, and laminitis) occurring in a period from the day of calving until 10 days post-calving.

Some of the physiological phenomena which make the transition period such an important time from the point of view of dairy cow health include: (a) a decline in feed intake when the nutrient requirements for impending lactogenesis and gestation are increasing; (b) a decline in calcium status with the onset of lactation: (c) an increase in the production of reactive oxygen metabolites; (d) an altered rumen fermentation resulting in varying degrees of ruminal or metabolic acidosis, (e) an acutely negative energy balance in the earliest weeks of lactation; (f) a myriad of endocrine changes associated with the onset of parturition, lactogenesis and resumption of ovarian cyclicity. Apart from these physiological phenomena, dairy cows must cope with and adapt to: (a) group changes that are part of normal dairy management and lead to reestablishment of hierarchical dominance within a group of cows; (b) the removal of the calf and associated stress soon after parturition; and (c) changes of environment that often necessitate differences in behaviour associated with feed and water consumption.

When these issues are considered it is of no surprise that dairy cows succumb to most disease conditions in this period. Many of the metabolic disorders, such as hypocalcaemia and ketosis are associated with this period, as are some notable production diseases, such as retained placenta and displaced abomasum. Furthermore, dairy cows experience varying degrees of periparturient immunosuppression in this period. The metabolic disorders are of course directly related to nutritional status, while nutritional status has also been implicated in many production diseases, such as those mentioned previously. However, it is also the case that the degree of immunosuppression experienced by dairy cattle in the periparturient period is modulated by nutritional status, including energy balance (Grummer, 2008), hypocalcaemia (Ducusin *et al.*, 2003), antioxidant status (Spears and Weiss, 2008), and acid-base balance (Enemark, 2008). Therefore, there is a complicated but well documented link between nutritional status and immune status in dairy cattle in the periparturient period.

1.2. Cascade-like sequences of periparturient cow pathologies

Periparturient health disorders are rarely isolated events. In many cases, one primary periparturient health disorder will lead to a whole sequence of health and productivity distortions that involves different biological systems within the body and different periods of time in the production cycle of the cow. For example, elevated Non-Esterified Fatty Acids (NEFAs) concentrations in the prepartum period have been associated with an increased risk of displaced abomasum in early lactation (Le Blanc *et al.*, 2005) whilst dairy cows that experience clinical hypocalcaemia have been demonstrated to have a greater risk of clinical endometritis in early lactation (Whiteford and Sheldon, 2005).

Furthermore, over-conditioned dry cows are also more likely to suffer from hypocalcaemia, which will also exacerbate immunosuppression and may cause dystocia and retained placenta (Houe *et al.*, 2001). Because of these complicated cascade-like sequences, diseases of the transition cow regularly result in the occurrence of infectious diseases or other production diseases or metabolic disorders, reduce fertility, reduce milk production and increase lameness. It is often difficult to determine which of the periparturient health disorders is the primary or causative disorder and all that can be said with certainty is that these conditions are related to each other. It is for this reason that prevention of production diseases has consequences for dairy cow welfare and producer profitability long after the transition period ends.

This paper will consider the following issues with regard to the influence of periparturient nutrition on early lactation pathologies of the dairy cow:
- over-conditioning and fatty liver;
- energy balance;
- milk fever and subclinical hypocalcaemia;
- gastrointestinal tract disorders.

The aim of this paper is not to review each of these areas in detail but to provide the reader with a useful summary of the current knowledge, describe how each one links to other metabolic disorders and infectious disease and to discuss some useful aspects of prevention.

2. Over-conditioning and fatty liver

Fatty liver or hepatic lipidosis is a condition that arises in dairy cows due to the accumulation of triacylglycerol (TAG) in hepatocytes. The accumulation of TAG in the liver of dairy cows is normally greatest during the periparturient period when the mobilisation of adipose tissue in the form of NEFAs is occurring at a very high rate. There are only three possible fates for the metabolism of NEFAs in the dairy cow liver: (1) complete oxidation to CO_2, (2) re-esterification and export from the liver as part of TAG in the form of very low-density lipoproteins (VLDL), and (3) incomplete oxidation to form ketone bodies, such as acetoacetate or β-hydroxy butyrate (BHB). The uptake of NEFAs by the liver is directly proportional to the flow rate of blood through the organ and the concentration of NEFAs in the blood (Grummer, 2008). During the periparturient period NEFA concentration in peripheral blood is at its highest. This is largely due to (1) a decline in dry matter intake as parturition approaches and the negative energy balance associated with the periparturient and early lactation period, (2) the natural hormonal events associated with the onset of parturition and the subsequent lactation (Ingvartsen, 2006), and (3) greater incidences of infections of the reproductive tract and mammary gland that pertain to periparturient dairy cows. Hence liver TAG concentrations are usually most elevated at this time.

Bobe *et al.* (2004) defined different classes of fatty liver based on liver TAG as a proportion of wet weight. Normal liver was defined as having <1% TAG, mild fatty liver was defined as 1-5% TAG, moderate fatty liver was defined as 5-10% TAG, while severe fatty liver was defined as >10% TAG. In a review of the literature these authors found that 20 to 53% of dairy cows could be classed as suffering from moderate fatty liver, while 5 to 24% of dairy cows could be define as suffering from severe fatty liver.

Obesity has been considered as a very important risk factor for the development of fatty liver in the dairy cow (Bobe *et al.*, 2004), albeit that not all reports agree with this finding (Ametaj, 2005). Dairy cows that are over-conditioned (BCS ≥ 4 on a scale of 1-5) would appear to be more susceptible to the development of fatty liver. Some of the reasons for this include (1) the greater reduction in dry matter intake in the close-up dry period that has been recorded by Hayirli *et al.* (2002), (2) a lower postpartum dry matter intake and more severe negative energy balance for cows with BCS of 4.0 at calving in comparison to lower BCS cows for the first weeks of lactation (Alibrahim *et al.*, 2008), and (3) elevated concentrations of NEFA in the peripheral blood of obese dairy cows in the periparturient period. Further confirmation of this association between obesity and fatty liver may be taken from the elevated levels of glutamate dehydrogenase and bilirubin found in obese periparturient cows (BCS = 4.0 at calving, scale = 1 to 5) in comparison to herd mates with lower BCS at parturition (BCS = 3.25 at calving, scale = 1 to 5) (see Figure 1 and 2) (O'Grady *et al.*, 2008a).

2.1. Consequences of over-conditioning and fatty liver

At the cellular level fatty liver is associated with fatty cysts in liver parenchyma, increased volume of individual hepatocytes, mitochondrial damage and compression and decreased volume of various cellular organelles including nuclei and rough endoplasmic reticulum (Bobe *et al.*, 2004). These documented changes at cellular level could be expected to have major consequences on nutrient metabolism, when the central role of the liver is considered. Although decreased ureagenesis and elevated ammonia levels in peripheral blood have been reported to accompany fatty liver (Strang *et al.*, 1998) a reduced capacity of

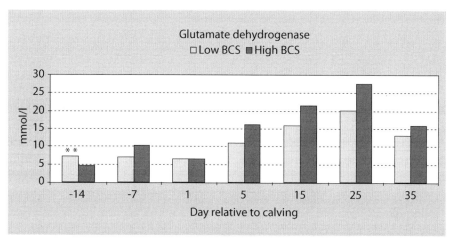

Figure 1. Glutamate dehydrogenase concentrations in peripheral blood of dairy cows with a high (4.0) and low (3.25) BCS at calving.
** Indicates significant difference between treatments at P<0.01.

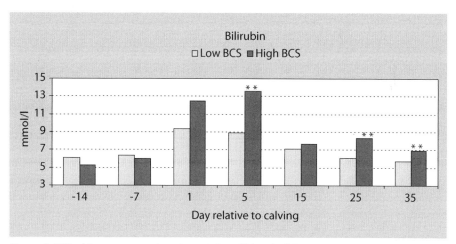

Figure 2. Bilirubin concentrations in peripheral blood of dairy cows with a high (4.0) and low (3.25) BCS at calving.
** Indicates significant difference between treatments at P<0.01.

hepatocytes for gluconeogensis has been demonstrated in some (Rukkwamsuk *et al.*, 1999; Murondoti *et al.*, 2004) but not in all reports (Grummer, 2008). These findings of a reduced capacity for gluconeogensis in dairy cows with fatty liver are consistent with the observations of Alibrahim *et al.* (2008) who reported lower glucose concentrations (*P*<0.05) in the peripheral blood of obese periparturient dairy cows (BCS = 4.0 at calving, scale = 1 to 5) in comparison to thinner herd mates in early lactation (BCS = 3.25 at calving, scale = 1 to 5). While some of this reduced glucose concentration was undoubtedly due to a lower feed intake, a reduced gluconeogenic capacity of hepatocytes is also likely to have contributed.

Fatty liver has often been associated with reduced reproductive performance of dairy cows (Jorristima *et al.*, 2000). While this association may be partly due to the increased severity of negative energy balance and reduced circulating levels of IGF-1 and glucose associated with fatty liver in dairy cows, other factors, such as delayed uterine involution and more severe and less responsive uterine infections following parturition have also been implicated (Bobe *et al.*, 2006). Further evidence of the effect of fatty liver and over-conditioning on reproductive performance is the lower early lactation insulin levels (*P*<0.05) recorded for obese cows at parturition in comparison to thinner herd mates (Alibrahim, unpublished results 2009). Both insulin and IGF-1 are required for resumption of ovulation in the postpartum period (Roche *et al.*, 2000). This is consistent with the findings of Mayne *et al.* (2002) who reported longer calving intervals for dairy herds that had a high average BCS in the dry period in comparison to herds with lower average BCS.

Both over-conditioning and fatty liver have been linked with other metabolic disorders, such as ketosis, displacement of the abomasum, milk fever, retained placenta, uterine infection, mastitis and difficult calving (Ingvartsen, 2006; Bobe *et al.*, 2006; Cameron *et al.*, 1998; Kaneene *et al.*, 1997; Zamet *et al.*, 1979a,b). While some of these conditions are undoubtedly consequences of over-conditioning, excessive adipose mobilisation and fatty liver, some which depress appetite in the periparturient period are likely to be predisposing factors (Ingvartsen, 2006). It is also interesting to note that ruminal acidosis and release of endotoxins by rumen bacteria has been implicated in the development of fatty liver (Ametaj, 2005). The clinical signs of the condition in cows with moderate or severe fatty liver vary from depression, lack of appetite and weight loss, reduced rumen motility (Ingvartsen, 2006) to, in severe cases, hepatic encephalopathy (ie., depressed conciousness, ataxia, somnolency, coma and death caused by liver or kidney failure or cardiac arrest) (Bobe *et al.*, 2004). The conflicting effects reported on milk yield (Ametaj, 2005; Grummer, 2008) may possibly be explained by the degree of fatty liver encountered. Ametaj (2005) reported negative effects of severe fatty liver on milk yield in the first six weeks of lactation. However, in our own studies dairy cows calving with a BCS of 4.0 (Scale = 1 to 5) recorded higher milk yield than those that calved with a BCS of 3.25 (Scale 1 to 5) (Alibrahim *et al.*, 2008).

Fatty liver has also been implicated in exacerbated immunosuppression in the periparturient period. Dairy cows with fatty liver have been demonstrated to have more prolonged periods of infectious diseases in the periparturient period. Bobe *et al.* (2006) reported that dairy cows with mild fatty liver had an increased number of days with elevated body temperature during the period 9-22 days postpartum in comparison to controls. Mild fatty liver was also associated with a higher incidence of mastitis, reduced reproductive performance (including reduced conception rate) and a longer period of time in negative energy balance. A reduced immune system competence for dairy cows suffering from fatty liver could be expected based on the findings of Hammon *et al.* (2006) who demonstrated reduced myeloperoxidase activity for polymorphonuclear leukocytes from dairy cows exposed to elevated NEFA in the periparturient period in comparison to controls. Furthermore, fatty liver resulted in a reduced expression of function-associated surface molecules on blood neutrophils and a reduced antibody-independent and -dependent cellular cytotoxicity of blood polymorphonuclear leukocytes in dairy cows (Zerbe *et al.*, 2000). Several other negative consequences of fatty liver on the immune system have been documented (Bobe *et al.*, 2004), as well as elevated concentrations of acute phase proteins haptoglobin and serum amyloid A in the first weeks following parturition (Ametaj, 2005).

2.2. Prevention

A recent review, which discusses the prevention of fatty liver has been published by Grummer (2008). Given the nature of this condition the principles of successful prevention are based on preventing over-conditioning (Bobe *et al.*, 2004; Ingvartsen, 2006), avoiding excessive adipose tissue mobilisation whether it is caused by severe reductions in feed intake or other conditions if ill health and assisting the export of TAG in VLDL from the liver (Grummer, 2008).

From the point of view of avoiding over-conditioning, dairy cows should calve down with a BCS of approximately 3.0 (Scale 1 to 5; Edmonson *et al.*, 1989). In order to achieve this target careful monitoring of BCS throughout the entire lactation cycle is warranted. While it could be argued that a higher BCS at calving may have advantages for milk yield (depending on the postpartum feeding regime employed), it is likely that cows with a BCS of 3.5 and above, will loose more BCS in the subsequent lactation (Buckley *et al.*, 2003), indicative of a more severe negative energy balance and thus predisposing these cows to metabolic disorders (mostly subclinical) and reduced fertility.

In terms of reducing adipose tissue mobilisation, recent research suggests a benefit from maintaining a marginally negative energy balance during the entire dry period as opposed to feeding a close-up dry cow diet of higher energy concentration derived from non-fibrous carbohydrate or fat (Dann *et al.*, 2005; Grummer, 2008). Supplementation of periparturient dairy cows with propylene glycol would appear to be a very satisfactory method of reducing adipose tissue mobilisation (Rizos *et al.*, 2004; Grummer, 2008). However, this is a time-consuming strategy as cows are usually dosed daily with the product. A recent experiment conducted at University College Dublin's Research farm has shown that there may be potential for the use of live yeast culture (*Saccharomyces cerivisae* CBS 493.94, Yea-Sacc[1026]) to reduce NEFA mobilisation in early lactation. In this experiment, supplementation with live yeast reduced NEFA concentrations in dairy cows at 25 days postpartum ($P=0.07$) (see Figure 3). A repeat study is currently ongoing to further investigate this interesting preliminary result. Bobe *et al.* (2004) has suggested that addition of glucose

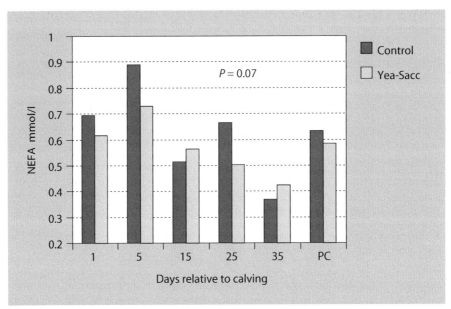

Figure 3. Non esterified fatty acid concentrations of peripheral blood for periparturient cows supplemented with Yea-Sacc and control cows.
PC: average for entire postcalving period.

precursors, such as propionate salts and glycerol may be an alternative to daily propylene glycol drenching.

In terms of aiding TAG excretion from the liver in the form of VLDL, Grummer (2008) has suggested that rumen protected-choline is a very useful product, while Bauchart *et al.*, (1998) has suggested that supplementation with rumen protected forms of lysine and methionine simultaneously may be of benefit due to the stimulation of hepatic apolipoprotein synthesis particularly apo B100 synthesis, which is essential for the excretion of TAG as part of VLDL. This latter observation is supported by the fact that dairy cows fed higher protein diets are less likely to suffer from fatty liver (Ingvartsen, 2006).

It is interesting to note that management of the transition cow in terms of avoiding stress (e.g., associated with group changes, environment changes, diet changes etc.) and treating any infectious conditions quickly could be just as important as nutrition in preventing fatty liver. One such management change is shortening or eliminating the dry period. This management change has proven useful in reducing the severity of NEB in early lactation and reducing TAG accumulation in liver (Grummer, 2008).

3. Negative energy balance

Negative energy balance in dairy cows arises when the energy ingested is insufficient to meet the energy requirements for maintenance and lactation or maintenance and gestation. While the negative energy balance associated with copious milk production is a problem for almost all cows in early lactation, not all cows are likely to experience negative energy balance pre-calving (Grummer, 2008). It is likely that those cows that experience negative energy balance pre-calving have experienced a large reduction in feed intake as parturition approaches (Hayirli *et al.*, 2002) or have been subjected to deliberate nutritional restriction in the dry period (McNamara *et al.*, 2003). Given that the energy requirements of most dry cows are quite easy to supply, most cows that do experience negative energy balance pre-calving are likely to do so in the last few days prior to parturition. There are many factors that may restrict feed intake more than normal at this time, such as dietary change, group changes, change of environment, over-conditioning and ill-health.

3.1. Consequences of negative energy balance

Many other periparturient cow health disorders may be associated with negative energy balance. These include, displaced abomasum (Le Blanc, 2005), retained placenta (Le Blanc, 2008), ketosis, fatty liver, immunosuppression (Hammon *et al.*, 2006) and reduced fertility performance. This review will focus briefly on immunosuppression and reduced fertility performance.

It has been well documented that negative energy balance (NEB) in early lactation causes reduced fertility performance (Roche *et al.*, 2000). The physiological basis for this association is as a reduced LH pulse frequency, reduced circulating concentrations of insulin and IGF-1, reduced secretion of oestradiol by ovarian follicles during NEB (Roche *et al.*, 2000) and deleterious effects of the metabolites NEFA and BHB together with low circulating glucose concentrations on oocyte development (Leroy *et al.*, 2005, 2006). It has often been demonstrated that where the severity of NEB is exacerbated, the resultant fertility performance is reduced (Buckley *et al.*, 2003). Hence, an important part of the nutritional management of dairy cows to ensure optimal fertility performance is to limit the extent and duration of NEB in early lactation.

Dairy cows that are subjected to excessive negative energy balance are also very likely to experience an exacerbated periparturient immunosuppression. This is likely one of the reasons that negative energy balance and retained placenta are associated (Le Blanc, 2008). Hammon *et al.* (2006) reported that dairy cows with lower dry matter intake during the periparturient period had lower capacity for phagocytosis by polymorphonuclear leukocytes as evidenced by reduced myeloperoxidase activity and cytochrome c reduction activity, in comparison to cows with higher dry matter intake. It is interesting that in this study, reduced dry matter intake and reduced neutrophil function were both associated with uterine health disorders. Further evidence of the effect of periparturient energy balance on immunosuppression may be taken from the study of Stabel *et al.* (2003). In this study, peripheral blood mononuclear cells from cows that were force-fed via a rumen cannula in the periparturient period demonstrated an increased secretion of immunoglobulin *in vitro* after parturition in comparison to control cows. However, other aspects of cell mediated immunity were not improved by force feeding in this study (Stabel *et al.*, 2003). Similar evidence of this effect of negative energy balance on immune system competence has been provided by Van Knegsel *et al.* (2007). In this experiment, it was demonstrated that the natural antibody concentration in plasma of periparturient dairy cows had a positive association with energy balance and dry matter intake.

3.2. Preventing negative energy balance

The two strategies that can be used to reduce the severity and duration of negative energy balance are (1) the reduction of milk energy output, and (2) the maximisation of feed intake. Various means of reducing milk energy output, such as reduced milking frequency, feeding low protein diets and reducing milk fat concentration have been employed in an attempt to improve energy balance in early lactation dairy cows. However, it can be argued that improving feed intake is a more acceptable means of improving energy balance especially as producer profitability will be heavily dependent on milk sales. Of course it is important that the extra feed intake is not simply matched with extra milk yield and some factors that are important in this regard include the lipogenic: glucogenic ratio of nutrients supplied by the diet (Gardener *et al.*, 1999), the protein concentration in the diet and the genotype of the cow.

One of the most fundamental aspects of preventing excessive negative energy balance pre- and post-calving is to avoid over-conditioning in the dry period and at calving. Several authors have reported that increased BCS at calving causes an increase in BCS loss in the following lactation (Garnsworthy and Webb, 1999; Alibrahim *et al.*, 2008). However, it is also important to appreciate that early lactation cows may experience excessive NEB in situations where over-conditioning at calving was not evident. These situations may arise due to problems, such as sub-optimal feed allowance for the milk yield potential of the herd, ill-health, poor feeding environment (inadequate trough space, poor grazing conditions), group stress, inadequate water supply or the provision of unpalatable diets.

While it is clear that elevated BCS at calving will exacerbate negative energy balance in early lactation, it would also appear that energy supply in relation to requirement has an important effect on early lactation cow energy balance. McNamara *et al.* (2003) demonstrated that feeding dairy cows below energy requirements for the last 4 weeks of the dry period reduced the severity and duration of the early lactation negative energy balance in comparison to cows fed above their energy requirements. It remains to be seen if this effect is independent of the effect of BCS at calving on early lactation energy balance.

It must be remembered that energy balance is at its nadir very early in lactation, very commonly in week one or two. Because of this periparturient cow health is very important for early lactation cow energy balance. Cows with periparturient health disorders, such as retained placenta, fat cow syndrome and milk fever have been reported to have a lower feed intake in the early postpartum period (Zamet *et al.*, 1979a,b). In support of this finding Bareille *et al.* (2003) reported that several periparturient health disorders, such as difficult calving, retained foetal membranes, milk fever, systemic mastitis, puerperal metritis and a foot lesion reduced feed intake. Several cytokines, including tumor-necrosis factor, interleukin 1 and interleukin 8, released as a component of the immune response to inflammatory conditions, such as mastitis and endometritis, may reduce feed intake (Ingvartsen and Andersen, 2000). Furthermore, Goff (2003) has extrapolated that the energy cost of an inflammatory response for a dairy cow of 600 kg body weight may amount to 4 Mcal per day and that this has deleterious consequences for cows already in negative energy balance. Thus it would appear that healthy periparturient cows are a prerequisite for avoiding excessive negative energy balance.

4. Milk fever and subclinical hypocalcaemia

Milk fever and subclinical hypocalcaemia are the most important macromineral disorders of transition dairy cows. Each case of milk fever has been recently estimated to cost €312 (Ryan and O'Grady, 2004), which includes an allowance for milk loss and for the cost of treatment. However, both milk fever and subclinical hypocalcaemia also predispose dairy cows to many other periparturient health disorders, which likely have a greater impact on dairy cow welfare and profitability than either condition alone. It has recently been estimated that between 3.5 and 7.5% of dairy cows succumb to clinical milk fever (De Garis and Lean, 2008). However, incidence rates as high as 34% have been reported in individual herds (Houe *et al.*, 2001) with incidence rates of this magnitude or even higher (up to 75%) encountered several times per year by the Dairy Herd Health Group at University College Dublin. Reported incidence rates for subclinical hypocalcaemia range from approximately 20 to 40% (Houe *et al.*, 2001) with incidence rates as high as 50% reported in multiparous US dairy cows (Goff, 2008). Interestingly Roche (2003) reported an incidence rate of 33% for subclinical hypocalcaemia for a group of grazing New Zealand dairy cows where milk fever incidence was only 4.8%. Therefore, although it is possible to maintain milk fever at incidence rates that are close to zero, it may not be possible to limit subclinical hypocalcaemia to such low incidence rates.

4.1. Consequences of milk fever and subclinical hypocalcaemia

Both milk fever and subclinical hypocalcaemia have been related to many other pathologies of the periparturient dairy cow. The biological phenomena that underpin these negative effects of milk fever would appear to be altered smooth and skeletal muscle function and an exacerbated immunosuppression in the periparturient period (Ducusin *et al.*, 2003; Kimura *et al.*, 2006). While it is not always possible to deduce the precise aetiological pathway by which milk fever and subclinical hypocalcaemia lead to a second periparturient health disorder in dairy cows, these proven phenomena should always be borne in mind.

It goes without saying that dairy cows immediately around the time of parturition require the optimal functioning of smooth and skeletal muscle. Several reports suggest that milk fever cows have an increased possibility of experiencing a difficult calving in comparison to normo-calcaemic cows. The magnitude of this increased likelihood has been reported to vary from 2.5 times more likely to as much as 6 times more likely (Curtis *et al.*,1983; Erb *et al.*, 1985; Correa *et al.*, 1993). Milk fever cows have also been reported to be more susceptible to uterine prolapse, with cows suffering from uterine prolapse demonstrating lower serum Ca concentration than cows that did not (Risco *et al.*, 1984). Interestingly, 19% of the cows in this study with uterine prolapse were reported to have severe or clinical hypocalcaemia (serum Ca <4 mg/dl), while a further 28% of the affected cows were classed as having moderate hypocalcaemia (serum Ca 4.1 to 6.0 mg/dl). This latter observation emphasises the relationship between subclinical hypocalcaemia and other periparturient health disorders.

When one considers the role of milk fever and subclinical hypocalcaemia in dystocia, it is not surprising at all to find that milk fever cows are more likely to suffer from retained placenta. Houe *et al.* (2001) have reported that milk fever cows are three times more likely to suffer from retained placenta, the direct effect of milk fever on retained placenta (leaving out any indirect effect arising from increased likelihood of dystocia) has been estimated to double the odds of retained placenta occurring (Erb *et al.*, 1985). It is also important to appreciate that subclinical, as well as clinical hypocalcaemia may predispose dairy cows to retained placenta. To this end, it has been reported that dairy cows suffering from retained placenta had a lower plasma Ca concentration at six hours after calving than normal cows, and that the level of Ca concentration recorded in plasma was consistent with subclinical and not clinical hypocalcaemia (Melendez *et al.*, 2004). Since it has been suggested that it is unlikely that lack of uterine contractility is a significant factor for the retention of foetal membranes (Le Blanc, 2008), the most likely explanation for this effect is the negative effect of hypocalcaemia on the immune system of the periparturient cow. When this effect of hypocalcaemia on the immune system is appreciated together with the negative effects on dystocia and retained placenta it is of no surprise that higher rates of clinical endometritis have been reported in milk fever cows in comparison to normal cows at around three weeks postpartum (Whiteford and Sheldon, 2005).

Milk fever has been reported to cause lower reproductive performance in dairy cows because of its effect on uterine muscle function, slower uterine involution (Borsberry and Dobson, 1989) and reduced blood flow to the ovaries (Jonsson and Daniel, 1997). It must also be appreciated that much of the effect of hypocalcaemia on fertility is an indirect effect mediated through dystocia, retained placenta and endometritis. This effect of milk fever on fertility has been reported to increase the number of services per conception (1.7 vs. 1.2), increase calving to first service interval (68 vs. 61 days) and increase calving to conception interval (88 vs. 76 days) for milk fever cows, in five UK dairy herds with an incidence rate of clinical milk fever of 7.5% (Borsbery and Dobson, 1989). The effect of hypocalcaemia on delayed uterine involution has been documented by Whiteford and Sheldon (2005) who reported that cows with milk fever had a greater diameter of the gravid uterine horn and non-gravid uterine horn between 15 and 45 days postpartum (indicative of slower uterine involution), and a significantly reduced likelihood of having a corpus luteum (indicative of the first postpartum ovulation) than normal cows. Furthermore, Kamgarpour *et al.* (1999) reported that subclinically hypocalcaemic cows have fewer ovulatory sized follicles at days 15, 30 and 45 postpartum and smaller follicles at first ovulation than normal cows. Thus it is not just the clinical cases that will have a reduced fertility performance.

Dairy cows that suffer from milk fever have been reported to be up to eight times more likely to develop mastitis in the subsequent lactation (Curtis *et al.*, 1983). The reasons for this are likely the combined effects of a reduction in teat sphincter muscle function and an exacerbated immunosuppression for periparturient cows with milk fever. It has been recently demonstrated that hypocalcaemia is associated with reduced intracellular Ca stores in peripheral blood mononuclear cells and that this exacerbates periparturient immunosuppression (Kimura *et al.*, 2006). A reduction in phagocytotic capacity by polymorphonuclear leukocytes of milk fever cows has also been demonstrated by Ducusin *et al.* (2003). The secretion of cortisol is believed to be an important reason for the suppressed immunity experienced by periparturient dairy cows. It has been demonstrated that both milk fever and subclinical hypocalcaemia cause an increase in the normal cortisol response at parturition (Horst and Jorgensen, 1982).

Perhaps the clearest demonstration of how hypocalcaemia can affect muscle function is the effect demonstrated on the frequency and amplitude of reticulorumen motility (Jorgensen *et al.*, 1998). This reduction in reticulorumen function may well affect the clearance rate of gastrointestinal tract contents and reduce feed intake as a result. Thus it is of no surprise that milk fever has been reported to have a relatively large negative effect on feed intake in dairy cows (Bareille *et al.*, 2003). In this publication, the effect of milk fever on feed intake was larger than the effect of a foot lesion or puerperal metritis. Given that subclinical hypocalcaemia may last for the first 10 days of the lactation, it is to be expected that cows suffering from hypocalcaemia will have a more severe negative energy balance than healthy cows. It is thus of no surprise that milk fever cows have been reported to have an increased likelihood of ketosis (Houe *et al.*, 2001).

Finally cows that suffer from milk fever and subclinical hypocalcaemia have been reported to have a higher incidence of displaced abomasum. It has been suggested that this effect may be caused by reduced motility and strength of abomasal contractions which in turn leads to abomasal atony and distension of the abomasum (Goff, 2003). However, it is perhaps just as likely that this association is due to reduced feed intake and higher incidence rates of ketosis, both of which have been related to milk fever (Houe *et al.*, 2001; Bareille *et al.*, 2003). This example serves to highlight the complicated web of interrelationship that connects periparturient diseases of the dairy cow.

4.2. Prevention of milk fever and subclinical hypocalcaemia

Many excellent reviews have recently been written about the prevention of milk fever and subclinical hypocalcaemia in dairy cows (Goff, 2008; DeGaris and Lean, 2008; Horst *et al.*, 1997). While a detailed review of prevention strategies is outside of the scope of this review, a pertinent summary of control principles and some recent information is presented.

It has long been known that over-conditioned dairy cows have an increased likelihood for the development of milk fever. This has been confirmed by Ostergaard *et al.* (2003) who reported that dairy cows that are over-conditioned at calving are up to four times more likely to develop milk fever. The reasons for this association between over-conditioning and milk fever may be (1) the extra Ca output in the milk of early lactation cows that are over-conditioned, (2) the reduced feed and hence mineral intake of over-conditioned cows in the close-up dry period, and (3) possibly a reduced capacity for liver and kidney tissue to produce sufficient quantities of the active form of vitamin-D3 in obese cows. It is interesting that this latter phenomenon has been demonstrated for liver tissue in obese human patients (Targher *et al.*, 2006).

Adequate magnesium (Mg) supplementation is vital for the prevention of milk fever. One of the most common findings of the University College Dublin Dairy Herd Health Group in milk fever problem herds is suboptimal magnesium status in dry cows. Magnesium plays a very important role in Ca metabolism, for example it is a key intermediate in the resorbtion of Ca from bone by parathyroid hormone. In a recent review, Mg supplementation was found to have the greatest influence amongst all dietary strategies for the prevention of milk fever (Lean *et al.*, 2006). Therefore, dietary Mg concentration for pregnant dairy cattle should be in the region of 0.4% of dry matter (DM) (Goff, 2004; Lean *et al.*, 2006). Lean *et al.* (2006) reported a reduction in milk fever incidence of 62% by increasing Mg supplementation from 0.3 to 0.4% of the diet.

Maintaining a negative Dietary Cation Anion Difference (DCAD) ((Na+K) – (Cl+S)) in close-up dry cow diets has long been recognised as an effective way to prevent milk fever. Block (1996) demonstrated a significant reduction in milk fever incidence using this method. The criteria for dietary evaluation using this method are: (1) achieving a DCAD of between -100 to -200 meq/kg of DM in the close-up dry cow diet (Goff and Horst, 1997); (2) maintenance of a dietary Ca concentration of approximately 1.2% (Oetzel *et al.*, 1988); and (3) that the urine pH of the cows fed this diet for several days demonstrates that sufficient metabolic acidosis has been achieved (i.e. urine pH should be in the range 6.0 to 6.8). In practical terms it can be very difficult to achieve a sufficiently negative DCAD where the potassium (K) concentration of the basal forage is >1.8% (Goff, 2008). However, even if the negative DCAD target cannot be met, it is likely that reducing DCAD and dietary K will have a positive effect on milk fever incidence in this situation (Lean *et al.*, 2006). Where dietary K concentrations are high to begin with, the positive effects of reducing dietary K on milk fever incidence likely lie in the reduced DCAD achieved and because K prevents Mg absorption from the gastrointestinal tract. It is interesting that Goff (2008) states that the key to milk fever prevention is to keep dietary K values close to 1.0% of DM, while the key to subclinical hypocalcaemia prevention is to add Cl to the diet to a level 0.5% below the K concentration.

Restricting Ca in the dry cow diet has classically been suggested as a means of milk fever prevention. This strategy works by causing an elevation in the levels of parathyroid hormone and activated vitamin-D3 in circulation before parturition. The net effect is that the normal 24 -48 hour delay in the response of these key regulators of Ca metabolism is avoided and Ca metabolism is primed for rapid mobilisation of Ca from bone and absorption for the gastrointestinal tract. However, in practice very low levels of Ca need to be fed to achieve this effect (<30 g per day) and it may be necessary to use Ca binders to achieve a prepartum hypocalcaemia and the desired effect on Ca metabolism (Goff, 2008). The addition of the Ca binders has been demonstrated to have a positive effect on milk fever incidence in dairy herds (Wilson, 2001).

Other means of milk fever prevention used frequently include, dosing cows with vitamin D products prepartum, or dosing with Ca at parturition. However, both are problematic. With regard to dosing with vitamin D products, the problems include the requirement for accurate prediction of calving dates, the need for repeat dosages should calving day be inaccurately predicted, the suppression of endogenous parathyroid hormone and vitamin-D3 unless slow withdrawal of the product happens after parturition and a greater likelihood of reoccurrence of milk fever 10 to 14 days postpartum. For Ca supplementation at parturition, most of the problems stem from the fact that intra-venous, oral and bolus preparations provide an elevated blood Ca status for a very short period (in some cases as little as 4 hours). While these products may be used to avoid milk fever, cows may still relapse into subclinical hypocalcaemia for first days of the lactation unless repeat doses are given at short time intervals.

5. Gastrointestinal tract disorders

5.1. Sub-acute ruminal acidosis (SARA)

At herd level, sub-acute ruminal acidosis may be defined as a rumen pH of less than 5.5 at a defined interval (typically 2 to 8 hours) after new feed allowance in 33% or more of 12 cows subjected to rumen pH sampling by rumenocentesis in an eligible group (Garret, 1996; Oetzel, 2003). In confined herds in the USA it has been reported that 19% of early lactation cows and 26% of mid lactation cows suffer from SARA, with 40% of cows affected in one third of the herds (Garret *et al.*, 1997). A similar report from Germany and the Netherlands indicated a slightly lower incidence rate of 11% for early lactation dairy cows and 18% for mid lactation dairy cows. For pasture fed herds, a lower incidence rate of 11% has been reported for Irish herds in mid-lactation (O'Grady *et al.*, 2008b) with a similar incidence rate of 10% reported in Australian herds (Bramley *et al.* 2006). The economic consequences of SARA have been estimated at a cost of €277 per cow per year (Ryan and O'Grady, 2004) or $1.12 per affected cow per day (Enemark, 2008). Early lactation cows and cows at peak dry matter intake are most at risk from SARA; the early lactation cows are at higher risk due to reduced absorptive capacity of the rumen, poorly adapted rumen microflora, and the rapid introduction to energy dense diets (Dirksen *et al.*, 1985), while cows at peak dry matter intake are at increased risk due to the greater amount of acids produced in the rumen. While Oetzel (2005) reported a higher incidence of SARA in mid-lactation in comparison to early lactation dairy cows in the USA, the problem of low rumen pH in the early lactation period should not be ignored given the negative consequences reported (Donovan *et al.*, 2004).

5.1.1. Consequences of SARA

Sub-acute ruminal acidosis has been associated with other conditions of ill-health, such as laminitis (Donovan *et al.*, 2004), reduced and erratic feed intake (Garrett, 1996), low body condition score in lactating cows (Oetzel, 2000), low milk fat syndrome, caudal vena caval syndrome (Enemark, 2008), abomasal displacement/ulceration (Olson, 1991), rumenitis (Enemark, 2008), immunosuppression (Kleen *et al.*, 2003) and inflammation (Plaizier *et al.*, 2008). Several excellent reviews on the consequences of SARA have recently been published (Kleen *et al.*, 2003; Enemark, 2008). However, it is apparent that the consequences of SARA on dairy cow health and productivity are not the same in all circumstances. A reduction in milk yield by 2.7 kg per day together with reductions in milk fat percentage and protein percentage of 0.3 and 0.12%, respectively have been reported by Stone (1999). In contrast no effect of SARA on milk production was reported by O'Grady *et al.* (2008b) or Bramley *et al.* (2006). These differences in the observed consequences of SARA are likely to extend to other health parameters also. For example, Plaizier *et al.* (2008) have reported very different effects of SARA on dairy cow health depending on whether it was induced by feeding grains or by reducing dietary particle size. This group demonstrated that grain-induced SARA caused increased concentrations of the acute phase proteins serum amyloid-A and haptoglobin in blood, whereas SARA induced by reducing fibre particle size did not. These authors have also reported that grain-induced SARA reduced feed dry matter intake and that although SARA induced by particle size reduction resulted in broadly similar ruminal pH, VFA and osmolarity, dry matter intake was not reduced by SARA induced by reducing feed particle size. Therefore, it is becoming apparent that the effects of low rumen pH on feed intake, milk production and the immune system of the cow will differ depending on whether the SARA was grain-induced or particle size-induced.

There has been a good deal of research interest in the effect of changing the diet of the transition cow from the dry cow diet to the lactating cow diet on rumen conditions. It has been shown that introducing diets, which increase propionate and butyrate in the VFA help the proliferation of rumen papillae, which are important for ruminal VFA absorption and maintenance of rumen pH in an optimal range (Dirksen *et al.*, 1985). While not all publications have demonstrated beneficial consequences of trying to achieve rumen adaption before parturition (McNamara *et al.*, 2003), it has been demonstrated that changing from a low energy diet to a high energy diet abruptly at calving may result in increased incidence of low rumen pH and increased hoof scores indicative of lameness between 55 and 75 days in milk (Donovan *et al.*, 2004). Therefore, while the advantages of gradual dietary change for transition dairy cows are not always obvious, the negative consequences of rapid dietary change if they occur can have an impact on dairy cow health and productivity through lameness and possibly also reduced feed intake and altered immune system competence. However, these effects likely depend on the diet fed pre-calving, the cause of low rumen pH and concurrent challenges to the barrier function of ruminal epithelium (Plaizier *et al.*, 2008).

5.1.2. Preventing SARA

The maintenance of adequate concentrations of dietary fibre is central to the prevention of SARA. In particular, the maintenance of adequate concentrations of physically effective fibre that stimulate chewing is a necessity to maintain rumen pH within an optimal range (Mertens, 1997). Mulligan *et al.* (2006) summarised several suggested evaluation criteria for the assessment of dietary fibre levels. These include total dietary crude fibre in the range 15 to 17%, total dietary NDF in the range of 27 to 30% and dietary NDF from forage of 21% at a minimum. Kleen *et al.* (2003) recommended similar levels of dietary crude fibre (CF) concentrations of 18%. Recommendations for dietary particle size differ with Shaver (1997) recommending that 15 to 20% of forage particles should be >4 cm in length while Oetzel (2003) recommended 7% of dietary fibre particles >3.5 cm in length. Problems with lack of effective fibre to stimulate chewing and salivary flow are associated with low concentrations of long forages while problems of unwanted diet sorting arise if excessive concentrations of forage particles are too long. Apart from dietary recommendations for minimum levels of fibre to prevent SARA, feeding errors, abrupt dietary change, irregular feeding patterns, excessive feeding at individual meals in component fed herds, aggressive feeding behaviour and poor feeding environment must always be considered as risk factors for SARA.

Enemark (2008) has recommended that transition cow dietary adjustment should take place over 4 to 6 weeks. This recommendation is supported by Kleen *et al.* (2003) who reported that the bacteriological changes associated with diet change are likely to take place within 3 weeks but that a further period is necessary for adjustment of rumen papillae. However, the consequences of abrupt dietary change are likely to differ between diets and may depend on the previous diet fed. While it is clear that abrupt dietary change has negative consequences in some cases (Donovan *et al.*, 2004) it is not clear if this is the case in all circumstances.

Other means of preventing SARA include the feeding of buffers and direct feed microbials. The use of buffer products, such as sodium bicarbonate has been found to have a positive effect on milk yield and feed intake in some studies (Erdman, 1988). Thus buffer products especially sodium bicarbonate may confer advantages where high levels of dietary starch and sugars and low levels of physically effective fibre are fed. The use of direct feed microbials, such as *Saccharomyces cerevisae* and *Lactobacillus plantarum* and *Enterococcus faeium* has been shown to improve productivity in early lactation cows in some studies (Nocek and Klautz, 2006) but not in others (Beauchamin *et al.*, 2003).

5.2. Displaced abomasum

Displaced abomasum is often a consequence of another periparturient health disorder of dairy cows. Between 80 and 90% of displaced abomasums that are diagnosed are diagnosed within one month of calving with the proportion that is estimated to occur within two weeks postpartum ranging from 55 to 85%. It has also been reported that up to 90% of the displacements that occur are left sided. The average incidence rate reported for left displaced abomasum (LDA) is 3.3%, with the incidence in individual herds reaching as high as 22% (Shaver, 1997). The average cost of displaced abomasum has been estimated at €515 (Ryan and O'Grady, 2004). Displacement of the abomasum would seem to be a consequence of several other periparturient health disorders. It has been reported that retained placenta, metritis and ketosis increase the chances of abomasal displacement with odds ratios of 6.8, 4.7 and 11.9 (Shaver, 1997). Furthermore, herds with higher incidences of milk fever and subclinical hypocalcaemia would appear to have a higher rate of abomasal displacement (Oetzel, 1996). While it has also been reported that herds with higher average blood NEFA prepartum or BHB postpartum have higher incidence of displaced abomasums (Le Blanc *et al.*, 2005). It is likely that most of these conditions increase the likelihood of displaced abomasum by causing the short-term reduction of feeding behaviour, which reduces rumen fill, or by causing disrupted feeding patterns. For milk fever and subclinical hypocalcaemia, reduced abomasal motility and reduced abomasal atony may also be implicated. The importance of rumen fill in the immediate periparturient period for the prevention of displaced abomasums cannot be underestimated. Coppock *et al.* (1972) reported that reducing dietary forage percentage from 75 to 30% prepartum increased the incidence of displaced abomasums from 0 to 36%. It must also be considered that excessive processing of dry cow diets may reduce rumen fill to such an extent that higher incidence rates of displaced abomasum result. Therefore, the key to preventing displaced abomasum is to try to maintain high rumen fill at parturition and in early lactation. It is thus important to prevent all periparturient health disorders that may reduce feed intake at this time, while both SARA and milk fever are likely related to displaced abomasum by more than one aetiological pathway.

6. Conclusions

Dairy cow nutrition has an important role to play in the prevention of periparturient health disorders. Failure to prevent periparturient health disorders has negative consequences for productivity, fertility, lameness and general health status that extend far beyond the periparturient period itself. Periparturient health disorders tend to be related to each other in complicated cascade-like sequences, such that the primary insult is often difficult to identify. Periparturient health disorders that have metabolic origins often lead to increased susceptibility to infectious diseases, such as mastitis or uterine infections. From the literature reviewed in this paper, and from the many problem herd investigations conducted by the Dairy Herd Health Group at University College Dublin, it is clear that appropriate nutritional management of the periparturient dairy cow must consider the following issues as a priority: (1) prevention of fatty liver and over-conditioning of dry cows, (2) prevention of excessively negative energy balance, (3) maintenance of an optimally functioning Ca metabolism, (4) maintenance of rumen pH within an optimal range, and (5) the provision of a full rumen at calving.

References

Alibrahim, R., P. Duffy, L. O'Grady, B. Beltman, A. Kelly, V.P. Gath, M.L. Doherty and Mulligan, F.J., 2008. The effect of body condition score at calving and supplementation with yeast on feed intake, blood metabolites and days to first ovulation in periparturiuent dairy cows. In: *Proceedings of World Buiatrics Congress*, Budapest, 6-11 July 2008, p. 7.

Ametaj, B.N., 2005. A new understanding of the causes of fatty liver in dairy cows. *Advances in Dairy Technology* **17**:97-112.

Bauchart, D., D. Durand, D. Gruffat and Y. Chillard, 1998. Mechanisms of liver steatosis in early lactation cows: effects of hepatoprotector agents. In: *Proceedings of The Cornell Nutrition Conference for Feed Manufacturers*, pp. 27-35.

Bareille N., F. Beaudeau, S. Billon, A. Robert and P. Faverdin, 2003. Effects of health disorders on feed intake and milk production in dairy cows. *Livestock Production Science* **83**:53-62.

Beauchamin, K.A., W.Z. Yang, D.P. Morgavi, G.R. Ghorbhani and W. Kautz, 2003. Effects of bacterial direct-fed microbials and yeast on site and extent of digestion, blood chemistry and subclinical rumen acidosis in feedlot cattle. *Journal of Animal Science* **81**:1628-1640.

Block, E., 1996. Anion-cation balance and its effect on the performance of ruminants. In: P.C. Garnsworthy and D.J.A. Cole (eds). *Recent Developments in Ruminant Nutrition 3*. Nottingham University Press, UK, pp. 323-340.

Bobe,, G., J.W. Young and D.C. Beitz, 2004. Pathology, etiology, prevention and treatment of fatty liver in dairy cows. *Journal of Dairy Science* **87**:3105-3124.

Bobe, G., B.N. Ametaj, D.C. Nafikov, D.C. Beitz and J.W. Young, 2006. Relationships between fatty liver and health and reporductive peroformance in Holstein cows. In Joshi, N.P. and Herdt, T.H., (eds.). *Production diseases in farm animals*. Proceedings of 12th International Conference. Wageningen Academic Publishers, Wageningen, the Netherlands, p. 154.

Borsberry, S. and H. Dobson, 1989. Periparturient diseases and their effect on reproductive performance in five dairy herds. *Veterinary Record*. **124**:217-219.

Bramley, E., I.J. Lean, W.J. Fulkerson, M.A. Stevenson, A.R. Rabiee and N.D. Costa, 2008. The definition of acidosis in dairy herds predominantly fed on pasture and concentrates. *Journal of Dairy Science*. **91**:308-321.

Buckley, F., K. O'Sullivan, J.F. Mee, R.D. Evans, and P. Dillon, 2003. Relationships among milk yield, body condition, cow weight and reproduction in Spring-Calved Holstein-Friesians. *Journal of Dairy Science* **86**:2308-2319.

Cameron, R.E.B., P.B. Dyk, T.H. Herdt, J.B. Kaneene, R. Miller, H.F. Bucholtz, J.S. Liesman, M.J. VandeHaar and R.S. Emery, 1998. Dry cow diet, management, and energy balance as risk factors for displaced abomasums in high producing dairy herds. *Journal of Dairy Science* **74**:1321-1326.

Coppock, C.E., C.H. Noller, S.A. Wolfe, C.J. Callahan and J.S. Baker, 1972. Effect of forage: concentrate ratio in complete feeds fed adlibitum on feed intake prepartum and the occurrence of abomasal displacement in dairy cows. *Journal of Dairy Science* **55**:783-789.

Correa, M.T., H. Erb and J. Scarlett, 1993. Path analysis for seven postpartum disorders in Holstein cows. *Journal of Dairy Science* **76**:1305-1312.

Curtis, C.R., H.N. Erb, C.J. Sniffen, R.D. Smith, P.A. Powers, M.C. Smith, M.E. White, R.B. Hilman and E.J. Pearson, 1983. Association of parturient hypocalcaemia with eight periparturient disorders in Holstein cows. *Journal of The American Veterinary Medical Association* **183**:559-561.

Dann, H.M., D.E. Morin, G.A. Bollero, M.R. Murphy and J.K. Drackley, 2005. Prepartum intake, postpartum induction of ketosis and periparturient disorders affect the metabolic status of dairy cows. *Journal of Dairy Science* **88**:3249-3264.

De Garis, P.J. and I.J. Lean, 2008. Milk fever in dairy cows a review of pathophysiology and control principles. *Veterinary Journal* **176**:58-69.

Dirksen, G.U., H.G. Liebich and E. Mayer, 1985. Adaptive changes of the ruminal mucosa and their functional and clinical significance. *Bovine Practitioner* **20**:116-120.

Donovan, G.A., C.A. Risco, G.M. DeChant Temple, T.Q. Tran and H.H. Van Horn, 2004. Influence of transition diets on occurrence of subclinical laminitis in Holstein dairy cows. *Journal of Dairy Science* **87**:73-84.

Drackley, J.K., 1999. Biology of dairy cows during the transition period: the final frontier. *Journal of Dairy Science* **82**:2259-2273.

Ducusin, R.J., Y. Uzuka, E. Satoh, M. Otani, M. Nishimura, S. Tanabe and T. Sarashina, 2003. Effects of extracellular Ca2+ on phagocytosis and intracellular Ca2+ concentrations in polymorphonuclear leukocytes of postpartum dairy cows. *Research in Veterinary Science* **75**:27-32.

Edmondson, A.J., I.J. Lean, L.D. Weaver, T. Farver and G. Webster, 1989. A body condition scoring chart for Holstein dairy cows. *Journal of Dairy Science* **72**:68-78.

Enemark, J.M.D., 2008. The monitoring, prevention of subacute ruminal acidosis: a review. *Veterinary Journal* **176**:32-43.

Erb, H.N., R.D. Smith, P.A. Oltenacu, C.L. Guard, R.B. Hilman, P.A. Powers, M.C. Smith and M.E. White, 1985. Path model of reproductive disorders and performance, milk fever, mastitis, milk yield and culling in Holstein cows. *Journal of Dairy Science* **68**:3337-3349.

Erdman, R.A., 1988. Dietary buffering requirements of the lactation cow: a review. *Journal of Dairy Science* **71**:3246-3266.

Gardener, N.H., C.K. Reynolds, R.H. Phipps, A.K. Jones and D.E. Beever, 1999. Effects of different diet supplements in the pre- and postpartum period on reproductive performance in the dairy cow. In: Diskin, M.G. (Ed.), *Fertility in the high producing dairy cow*. BSAS Occasional Symposium No. 26, pp. 313-322.

Garnsworthy, P.C. and R. Webb, 1999. The influence of nutrition on fertility in dairy cows. In: J. Wiseman and P.C. Garnsworthy (Eds.). *Recent developments in ruminant nutrition 4*. Nottingham University Press, pp. 499-516.

Garrett, E., 1996. Subacute rumen acidosis. Clinical signs and diagnosis in dairy herds. *Large Animal Veterinarian* 11:6-10.

Garrett, E.F., K.V. Nordlund, W.J. Goodger and G.R. Oetzel, 1997. A cross-sectional field study investigating the effect of periparturient dietary management on ruminal pH in early lactation dairy cows. *Journal of Dairy Science* 80(Suppl. 1):169.

Goff, J.P., 2003. Managing the transition cow – considerations for optimising energy and protein balance and immune function: *Cattle Practice* 11(2):51-63.

Goff, J.P., 2004. Macromineral disorders of the transition cow. *Veterinary Clinics Food Animal Practice* 20:471-494.

Goff, J.P., 2008. The monitoring, prevention and treatment of milk fever and subclinical hypocalcaemia in dairy cows. *Veterinary Journal* 176:50-57.

Goff, J.P. and R.L. Horst, 1997. Effects of the addition of potassium or sodium, but not calcium, to prepartum rations on milk fever in dairy cows. *Journal of Dairy Science* 80:176-186.

Grummer, R.R., 1995. Impact of changes in organic nutrient metabolism on feeding the transition cow. *Journal of Animal Science* 73:2820-2833.

Grummer, R.R., 2008. Nutritional and management strategies for the prevention of fatty liver in dairy cattle. *Veterinary Journal* 176:10-20.

Hammon, D.S., I.M. Evjen, T.R. Dhiman, J.P. Goff and J.L. Walters, 2007. Neutrophil function and energy status in Holstein cows with uterine health disorders. *Veterinary Immunology and Immunopathology* 113:21-29.

Hayirli, A., R.R. Grummer, E.V. Nordheim and P.M. Crump, 2002. Animal and dietary factors affecting feed intake during the prefresh transition period in Holsteins. *Journal of Dairy Science* 85:3430-3443.

Horst, R.L. and R.J. Jorgensen, 1982. Elevated plasma cortisol during induced and spontaneous hypocalcaemia in ruminants. *Journal of Dairy Science* 65:2332.

Horst, R.L., J.P. Goff, T.A. Reinhardt and D.R. Buxton, 1997. Strategies for preventing milk fever in dairy cattle. *Journal of Dairy Science* 80:1269-1280.

Houe, H., S. Ostergaard, T. Thilsing-Hansen, R.J. Jorgensen, T. Larsen, J.T. Sorensen, J.F. Agger and J.Y. Blom, 2001. Milk fever and subclinical hypocalcaemia – an evaluation of parameters on incidence risk, diagnosis, risk factors and biological effects as input for a decision support system for disease control. *Acta Veterinaria Scandinavicia* 42:1-29.

Ingvartsen, K.L., 2006. Feeding and management related diseases in the transition cow. Physiological adaptions around calving and strategies to reduce feeding related diseases. *Animal Feed Science and Technology* **126**:175-213.

Ingvartsen, K.L. and J.B. Andersen, 2000. Integration of metabolism and intake regulation: a review focusing on periparturient animals. *Journal of Dairy Science* **83**:1573-1597.

Ingvartsen, K.L., R.J. Dewhurst and N.C. Friggens, 2003. On the relationship between lactational performance and health: is it yield or metabolic imbalance that cause production diseases in dairy cattle? A position paper. *Livestock Production Science* **83**:277-308.

Jonsson, N.N. and R.C.W. Daniel, 1997. Effect of hypocalcaemia in blood flow to the ovaries of sheep. *Journal of the American Veterinary Medical Association* **44**:281-287.

Jorgensen, R.J., N.R. Nyengaard, S. Hara, J.M. Enemark and P.H. Andersen, 1998. Rumen motility during induced hyper- and hypocalcaemia. *Acta Veterinaria Scandinavicia* **39**:331-338.

Jorristima, R.H., H. Jorristima, Y.H. Schukken and G.H. Wentink, 2000. Relationships between fatty liver and fertility and some periparturient diseases in commercial Dutch dairy herds. *Theriogenology* **54**:1065-1074.

Kamgarpour, R., R.C.W. Daniel, D.C. Fenwick, K. McGuigan and G. Murphy, 1999. Postpartum subclinical hypocalcaemia and effects on ovarian function and uterine involution in a dairy herd. *Veterinary Journal* **158**:59-67.

Kimura, K., T.A. Reinhardt and J.P. Goff, 2006. Parturition and hypocalcaemia blunts calcium signals and immune cells of dairy cattle. *Journal of Dairy Science* **89**:2588-2595.

Kaneene, J.B., R. Miller, T.H. Herdt and J.C. Gardiner, 1997. The association of serum nonesterified fatty acids and cholesterol, management and feeding practices with peripartum disease in dairy cows. *Preventative Veterinary Medicine* **31**:59-72.

Kleen, J.L., G.A. Hooijer, J. Rehage and J.P.T.M. Noordhuizen, 2003. Subacute Ruminal Acidosis (SARA): a review. *Journal of Veterinary Medicine A* **50**:406-414.

Le Blanc, S.J., K.E. Leslie and T.F. Duffield, 2005. Metabolic predictors of displaced abomasums in dairy cattle. *Journal of Dairy Science* **88**:159-170.

Le Blanc, S.J., 2008. Postpartum uterine disease and dairy herd reproductive performance: a review. *Veterinary Journal* **176**:102-114.

Lean, I.J., P.J. DeGaris, D.M. McNeil and E. Block, 2006. Hypocalcemia in dairy cows: meta-analysis and dietary cation anion difference theory revisited. *Journal of Dairy Science* **89**:669-684.

Leroy, J.L., T. Vanholder, B. Mateusen, A. Christophe, G. Opsomer, A. De Kruif, G. Genicot and A. Van Soom, 2005. Non-esterified fatty acids in follicular fluid of dairy cows and their effect on developmental capacity of bovine oocytes in vitro. *Reproduction* **130**:485-495.

Leroy, J.L.M., T. Vanholder, G. Opsomer, A. Van Soom and A. De Kruif, 2006 The in vitro development of bovine oocytes after maturation in glucose and beta-hydroxybutyrate concentrations associated with negative energy balance in dairy cows. *Reproduction in Domestic Animals* **41**(2):119-123.

McNamara, S., J.J. Murphy, M. Rath and F.P. O'Mara, 2003. Effects of different transition diets on energy balance, blood metabolites and reproductive performance in dairy cows. *Livestock Production Science* **84**:195-206.

Melendez, P., G.A. Donovan, C.A. Risco and J.P. Goff, 2004. *American Journal of Veterinary Research* **65**:1071-7076.

Mayne, C.S., M.A. McCoy, S.D. Lennox, D.R. Mackey, M. Verner, D.C. Catney, W.J. McCaughey, A.R.G. Wylie, B.W. Kennedy and F.J. Gordon, 2002. Fertility of dairy cows in Northern Ireland. *Veterinary Record* 150:707-713.

Mertens, D.R., 1997. Creating a system for meeting the fibre requirements of dairy cows. *Journal of Dairy Science* **80**:1463-1481.

Mulligan, F.J., L.O. O'Grady, D.A. Rice and M.L. Doherty, 2006. A herd health approach to dairy cow nutrition and production diseases of the transition cow. *Animal Reproduction Science* **96**:331-353.

Murondoti, A., R. Jorristma, A.C. Beynen, T. Wensing and M.J. Geelen, 2004. Activities of the enzymes of hepatic gluconeogenesis in periparturient dairy cows with induced fatty liver. *Journal of Dairy Research* **71**:129-134.

Nocek, J.E. and W.P. Klautz, 2006. Direct-fed microbial supplementation on ruminal digestion health and performance of pre- and postpartum dairy cattle. *Journal of Dairy Science* **89**:260-266.

O'Grady, L., R. Alibrahim, V.P. Gath, M.L. Doherty and F.J. Mulligan, 2008a. Body condition score at calving and supplementation with yeast affect blood mineral and liver enzyme concentrations in peripheral blood of periparturient dairy cows. In: *Proceedings of World Buiatrics Congress*, Budapest, 6-11 July 2008, p. 42.

O'Grady, L., M.L. Doherty and F.J. Mulligan, 2008b. Sub acute ruminal acidosis (SARA) in grazing Irish dairy cows. *Veterinary Journal* **176**:44-49.

Oetzel, G.R., J.D. Olsson, C.R. Curtisand and M.J. Fettman, 1988. Ammonium chloride and ammonium sulphate for the prevention of parturient paresis in dairy cattle. *Journal of Dairy Science* **71**:3302-3309.

Oetzel, G.R., 1996. Effect of calcium chloride gel treatment in dairy cows on incidence of periparturient diseases. *Journal of American Veterinary Medical* Association **209**(5):958-961.

Oetzel, G.R., 2000. Clinical aspects of ruminal acidosis in dairy cattle. In: *Proceedings, 33rd Annual Meeting of the American Association of Bovine Practitioners*, Rapid City, SD, USA, pp. 46-53.

Oetzel, G.R., 2003. Subacute ruminal acidosis in dairy cattle. *Advances in Dairy Technology* **15**:307-317.

Oetzel, G.R., 2005. Applied aspects of ruminal acidosis induction and prevention. *Journal of Dairy Science* **88**(Suppl 1):643.

Ostergaard, S., J.T. Sorensen and H. Houe, 2003. A stochastic model simulating milk fever in a dairy herd. *Preventative Veterinary Medicine* **58**:125-143.

Olson, J.D., 1991. Relationship of nutrition to abomasal displacement and parturient paresis. *Bovine Practice* **26**:88-91.

Plaizier, J.C., D.O. Krause, G.N. Gozho and B.W. McBride, 2008. Sub acute ruminal acidosis in dairy cows: The physiological causes, incidence and consequences. *Veterinary Journal* **176**:21-31.

Risco, C.A., J.P. Reynolds and D. Hird, 1984. Uterine prolapse and hypocalcaemia in dairy cows. *Journal of the American Veterinary Medicine Association* **185**:1517-1519.

Rizos, D., W. Griffin, P. Duffy, C. Quinn, F.J. Mulligan, J.F. Roche, M.P. Boland and P. Lonergan, 2004. The effect of feeding propylene glycol to dairy cows during the early postpartum on insulin concentration and the relationship with oocyte developmental competence. *Reproduction Fertility and Development* **16**(1-2):262.

Roche, J.F., D. Mackey and M.D. Diskin, 2000. Reproductive management of postpartum cows. *Animal Reproduction Science* **60-61**:703-712.

Roche, J.R., 2003. The incidence and control of hypocalcaemia in pasture-based systems. *Acta Veterinaria Scandinavicia* **97**(1):141-144.

Rukkwamsuk, T., T. Wensing and M.J.H. Geelen, 1999. Effect of fatty liver on hepatic gluconeogenesis in periparturient dairy cows. *Journal of Dairy Science* **82**:500-505.

Ryan, E.G. and L. O'Grady, 2004. The economics of infectious and production diseases in dairy herds. In: *Herd health planning*. Veterinary Ireland Publishers, pp. 3-50.

Shaver, R.D., 1997. Nutritional risk factors in the etiology of left displaced abomasums in dairy cows: a review. *Journal of Dairy Science* **80**:2449-2453.

Spears, J.W. and W.P. Weiss, 2008. Role of antioxidants and trace elements in health and immunity of transition dairy cows. *Veterinary Journal* **176**:70-76.

Stabel, J.R., J.P. Goff and K. Kimura, 2003. Effects of supplemental energy on metabolic and immune measurements in periparturient dairy cows with Johne's disease. *Journal of Dairy Science* **86**:3527-3535.

Stone, W.C., 1999. The effect of subclinical rumen acidosis on milk components. In. *Proceedings of Cornell Nutrition Conference for Feed Manufacturers*. Cornell University, Ithaca, NY. USA. pp. 40-46.

Strang, B.D., S.J. Bertics, R.R. Grummer and L.E. Armentano, 1998. Effect of long chain fatty acids on triglyceride accumulation, gluconeogenesis and ureagenesis in bovine hepatocytes. *Journal of Dairy Science* **81**:728-739.

Targher, G., L. Bertolini, L. Scala, M. Cigolini, L. Zenari, G. Falezza and G. Arcaro, 2006 Associations between serum 25-hydroxyvitamin D_3 concentrations and liver histology in patients with non-alcoholic fatty liver disease. *Nutrition, Metabolism and Cardiovascular Diseases* **17**(7):517-524.

Van Knegsel, A.T.M., G. De Vries Reilnigh, S. Meulenberg, H. Van den Brand, J. Dijkstra, B. Kemp and H.K. Parmentier, 2007. Natural antibodies related to energy balance in early lactation dairy cows. *Journal of Dairy Science* **90**:5490-5498.

Whiteford, L.C. and I.M. Sheldon, 2005. Association between clinical hypocalcaemia and postpartum endometritis. *Veterinary Record* **157**:202-204.

Wilson, G.F., 2001. A novel nutritional strategy to prevent milk fever and stimulate milk production in dairy cows. *New Zealand Veterinary Journal* **49**(2):78-80.

Zamet, C.N., V.F. Colenbrander, C.J. Callaghan, B.P. Chew, R.E. Erb and N.J. Moeller, 1979a. Variables associated with peripartum traits in dairy cows. I. Effect of dietary forages and disorders on voluntary intake of feed, body weight and milk yield. *Theriogenology* **11**:229-244.

Zamet, C.N., V.F. Colenbrander, C.J. Callaghan, B.P. Chew, R.E. Erb and N.J. Moeller, 1979b. Variables associated with peripartum traits in dairy cows. II. Interrelationships among disorders and their effects on intake of feed and reproductive efficiency. *Theriogenology* **11**:245-260.

Zerbe, H., N. Schneider, W. Leibold, T. Wensing, T.A.M. Kruip and H.J. Schubert, 2000. Altered functional and immunophenotypical properties of neutrophilil granulocytes in postpartum cows associated with fatty liver. *Theriogenology* **54**:771-786.

Nutritional impact on lameness in dairy cows

J.R. Scaife[1] and H. Galbraith[2]
[1]School of Equine and Animal Science, Writtle College, Lordship Road, Chelmsford, CM1 3RR, United Kingdom
[2]School of Biological Sciences, University of Aberdeen, 23 St Machar Drive, Aberdeen, AB24 3RY, United Kingdom

1. Introduction

It has been estimated that 60% of all animals in contemporary dairy herds are affected by lameness (Vermunt, 2004). The consequences of this painful condition can be poor reproductive performance and loss of milk yield. The multifactorial nature of the aetiology of lameness is well recognised (Figure 1) and in discussing the impact of nutrition on the occurrence of lameness in dairy cows, the contribution of housing environments and housing systems should not be overlooked. A comprehensive review of the influence of nutrition on claw composition and health has recently been published (Galbraith and Scaife, 2008).

In the dairy cow, the largest proportion of cases of lameness are located in the claws. The claws of all four feet can be affected by symptoms characteristic of infectious lameness, for example caused by digital dermatitis, and non-infectious lameness, typified by white line disease (WLD), sole ulcer and solar haemorrhage. However, it is the hind feet that are most commonly affected and the lateral claws, which are most likely to develop lesions and abnormalities and show clinical signs of damage. Approximately 75% of lameness is known to be associated with claw horn lesions (Logue *et al.*, 1993).

In describing the impact of nutrition on the incidence of lameness, it is important to consider the basic anatomy of the bovine claw and identify those components, which are most susceptible to dietary factors and disturbances in nutrient supply. There are clear implications for nutritional inputs, which are required to support tissue homeostasis and integrity of the claw. These include amino acids, proteins, carbohydrates, lipids, minerals and vitamins which contribute to anatomical structure and metabolic activity.

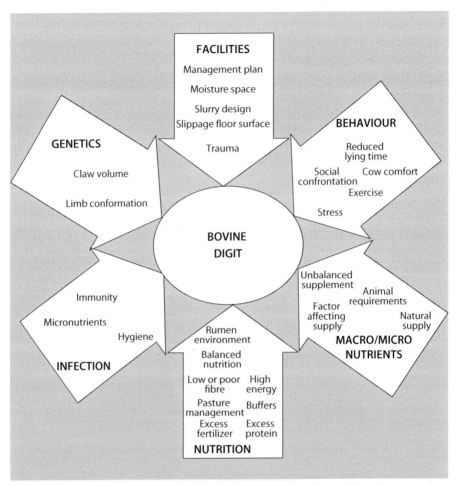

Figure 1. Multifactorial nature of the causes of lameness (Adapted from Greenough et al., *1997).*

2. Anatomy of the claw and biomechanical function

The basic anatomy of the bovine claw is shown in Figure 2. The primary function of the components of bovine claw is to transfer the body weight of the animal to the ground surface. This transfer is achieved by transmission of the mechanical forces incident upon the pedal bone to the hoof horn capsule. When viewed in saggital section, it can be seen that the pedal bone is suspended inside the horn capsule. Extensive study of the ultrastructure of the tissues linking the pedal bone to the hoof wall has shown the presence

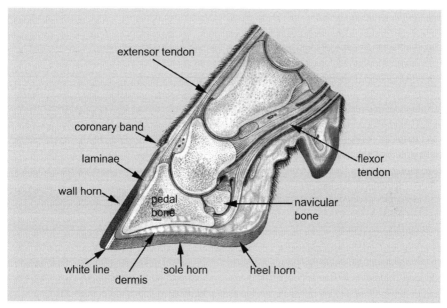

Figure 2. Structure of the bovine claw (Adapted from Budras and Wünsche, 2002).

of an intricate suspensory apparatus, which effectively holds the pedal bone suspended within the horn capsule.

The suspensory apparatus consists of an intricate system of laminae in the dermis and epidermis of the claw wall, which interdigitate to provide a strong yet flexible link between the pedal bone and the claw horn capsule (Figure 3). Beneath the pedal bone the underlying soft tissue has been shown to contain cylindrical pads of adipose tissue, referred to as digital cushions that protect the dermis and epidermis of the sole from mechanical damage caused by the pedal bone by acting as 'shock absorbers'. The role of the digital cushions has been likened to the structures incorporated into the sole of running shoes to lessen the impact of weight transfer to the ground (Lischer and Ossent, 2000). Reductions in the efficacy of the suspensory system in preventing the excessive impact of the pedal bone on dermal and epidermal soft tissue in sole and heel are considered a major cause of lesion formation. The solear and heel components of the horn capsule have an important role in protecting underlying soft tissue from the ground surface and thin soles (5 mm or less) have been associated with greater susceptibility to damage to underlying soft tissue (Van Amstel *et al.*, 2004). Loss of functionality in either the suspensory components of the claw

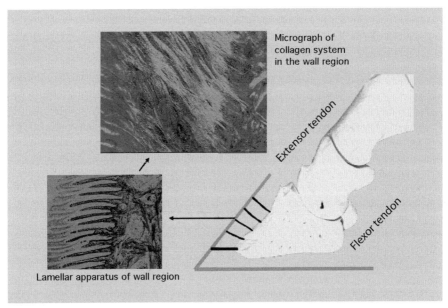

Micrograph of collagen system in the wall region

Extensor tendon

Flexor tendon

Lamellar apparatus of wall region

Figure 3. Suspensory apparatus of the bovine foot.

wall, or the digital cushions, or both can lead to increased pressure of the pedal bone on the corium and the development of sole ulcers.

3. Cell and molecular biology of horn production

Hoof horn is the end-product of a process of differentiation, keratinisation and cornification of epidermal cells which begin their journey to the outer surface of the horn capsule at the interface between the dermis and epidermis. These cells, 'keratinocytes', proliferate on a basement membrane which separates the dermis from the epidermis (Budras *et al.*, 1998; Galbraith *et al.*, 2006). The dermis is at the margins of vascularised tissues and a key factor associated with production of good quality hoof horn is the fact that the epidermis is avascular and keratinocytes receive nutrients, regulatory mitogens and morphogens across the basement membrane from the dermis. As a result, the biosynthetic activity of epidermal tissues and keratinocytes in particular is sensitive to changes in nutrient supply originating from variation in dietary supply of macro- and micro-nutrients or as a result of disruption of the blood supply to the dermis, which in turn will affect the supply of nutrients at the dermal/epidermal interface. In addition, it is generally accepted that dietary conditions which lead to the development of subacute rumen acidosis (SARA) can lead to changes in blood flow in the dermis and release of autolytic enzymes which reduce the physical strength of the suspensory apparatus causing the pedal bone to rotate and impact upon the soft tissues of the sole resulting in haemorrhage and lesion formation.

4. Dietary management and rumen acidosis

In general the mechanisms by which nutrition can affect the development of lameness in high yielding dairy cows are poorly understood. The physical characteristics of the diet, for example, wet versus dry feeds or complete (TMR) versus component feeding systems may influence the digestive process and the supply of nutrients. Similarly, the availability of feed, the timing of access to feeds and the amount of space allowed for feeding and rumination will affect the feeding pattern and activity level of individual cows in a herd. In addition, consideration must also be given to the relative contribution of the 'direct' effects of the diets in the context of the impact of diet on events in the rumen and the supply of nutrients to metabolically active tissues of the foot, and 'indirect' effects of the diets on activity levels in the cows, time spent eating and ruminating and the chemical composition and physical nature of slurry produced.

Dietary conditions, which lead to the development and persistence of subacute rumen acidosis (SARA) have received considerable attention in recent years although the link between events in the rumen and the development of laminitis or *pododermatitis aseptica diffusa* (PAD) in the bovine claw remain to be clearly established. The quantity and quality of individual nutrients in the diet has the potential to impact on the supply of key nutrients to the dermal/epidermal unit.

Nutritional and management changes made some time prior to calving may be considered as risk factors that influence the development of claw horn lesions (CHL) long before the clinical symptoms of lameness can be seen. Numerous studies have reported a higher incidence of CHL in animals fed a low dry matter fermented forage-based diet compared those fed a high dry matter unfermented forage diets (Offer *et al.*, 2003; Leach *et al.*, 2005). Observations have also been made, which suggest that the feeding of complete rations (TMRs) is less likely to lead to the development of SARA than the feeding of component diets and that refinement of the formulation and management of TMR feeding can contribute to a reduction in the incidence of this condition, which is associated with the development of PAD (Stone, 2004). The mechanisms by which these dietary factors influence the incidence of claw horn lesions remains to be determined in detail. It is clear that the diet has direct effects on digestive processes, which have consequences for nutrient supply and metabolic events relating to claw health. In addition, presentation, structure and composition of the diets can have indirect effects on the incidence of lameness by changing feeding behaviour, activity levels (ruminating/lying times) and the physical environment, for example the quantity and consistency of slurry.

Stone (2004) has reviewed a number of aspects of nutritional management that warrant attention in order to minimise the risk of acidosis. Factors, such as the amount of physically effective neutral detergent fibre in the ration, their rumen fermentabilities, predicted organic acid production and ratio to non-structural carbohydrate supply should be considered. Variability in the ration formulation and physical form can also result in changes in palatability and intake. Systems to ensure the uniformity of the ration presented to animals need to be in place and feed characteristics, such as fibre length, wetness of the ration and the frequency of feed pushups can be manipulated to minimise sorting.

While diets rich in highly fermentable carbohydrates increase milk production they also increase the risk of SARA, which is characterised by a prolonged period during which the rumen pH is between pH 5.2 and 5.6 (Owens *et al.*, 1998, Keunen *et al.*, 2002). Much attention has been paid recently to the causes and management of SARA and it is still widely accepted that as a consequence of the associated change in rumen environment, changes in the permeability characteristics of the rumen wall can result in the absorption of bioactive molecules with the ability to influence the microcirculation of the dermis of the hoof and reduce nutrient supply to the proliferating cells of the epidermis. In addition, and maybe as a consequence of the changes in microcirculation, the physical strength of the dermal/epidermal junction may be reduced by the activation of matrix metalloproteinases (MMPs) which weaken the suspensory components of the claw wall (Tarlton *et al.*, 2003). As a result the pedal bone rotates within the horn capsule causing compression of the soft epidermal tissue of the sole and heel eventually leading to lesion formation. Webster *et al.* (2005) has argued that the changes in the structural integrity of the claw horn are not caused by inflammation of the laminae but have a non-inflammatory basis due to enzyme-mediated changes in the connective tissue of the suspensory apparatus.

Work carried out as part of the EU Framework 5 LAMECOW project has provided some insight into the relationship between metabolic disturbances thought to be characteristic of SARA, and changes in integrity of the dermal/

epidermal junction of the claw. Using a novel *in vitro* model for organotypic cell culture and an isolated haematoperfused distal cow limb model, Mülling *et al.* (2006) recently provided evidence for the involvement of endotoxins, histamine and lactate as effector molecules in the claw and has proposed involvement of the inflammatory cytokine, interleukin 1 (IL1) in the regulation of cellular changes resulting in the release of keratinocyte growth factor, a potent mitogen, which stimulates the proliferation of basal epidermal cells. In addition, IL1 has the potential to activate MMPs resulting in the weakening of the laminae at the dermal/epidermal interface.

5. The impact of specific nutrients

Tomlinson *et al.* (2004) and Galbraith and Scaife (2008) suggested that nutrient supply was one of the factors, which influence the growth and development of the tissues of the bovine claw and identified a number of candidate nutrients. Maintaining a balanced supply of individual nutrients to the proliferating cells of the epidermis of the wall and sole of the claw is essential.

5.1. Protein and amino acids

The principle protein components of hoof horn are keratins which, along with certain keratin-associated proteins (KAPS), are characterised by relatively high content of the sulphur-containing amino acid cysteine. This amino acid is essential in the formation of disulphide bonds within and between the keratin molecules that constitute a large part of the filamentous proteinaceous structures of the cytoskeleton. Methionine is present in keratins at much lower concentrations and does not contribute directly to the formation of disulphide bonds, however, its dietary supply and availability in proliferating epidermal cells provide a mechanism through trans-sulphuration pathways for the synthesis of cysteine *in situ*. There is conflicting evidence that supplementation of diets with rumen protected, intestinally digestible L-methionine or its analogues may increase growth rates of hoof horn. Any clear benefits of such a strategy on the incidence of hoof lesions have yet to be demonstrated.

The extent to which dietary protein is responsible for causing laminitis or lameness still remains unclear. Livesey and Laven (2007) have recently reported some features of protein nutrition and claw horn health. It is apparent that protein makes up a significant part of the structure of the claw dermis and epidermis. In order to understand the appropriate dietary protein intake necessary for maintenance of the structural integrity of the hoof horn, it is imperative to consider the amino acid composition of the horn. Table 1 shows a comparison between some selected amino acid composition in horn and muscle tissues with those present in rumen microbial protein and some ruminant dietary protein sources as reported in Galbraith (1995) and Galbraith *et al.* (2006). The results show that of all of the amino acids, the proportion of cysteine from the ruminant feed sources is less (0.2-0.33) than that deposited in the horn samples studied. Methionine was also observed to be present to a significantly lower extent than cysteine.

Methionine is a nutritionally essential amino acid, which plays an important role in peptide translation and synthesis, methylation and synthesis of polyamines in addition to a role in the structure of horn proteins, although at a lower concentration than cysteine (Reis, 1989). Galbraith *et al.* (2006) reported that horn hardness was associated with the cysteine and methionine content of horn, being harder in the wall where the ratio of cysteine to methionine was higher than in the softer sole and heel horn. These results may suggest an increased expression of protein with high content of cysteine in the dorsal wall than solear horn. The fact that cysteine is an amino acid that is susceptible to oxidation has led to strategies to increase its supply indirectly by dietary supplementation with L-methionine or its analogues. This has been done both in rumen-protected, as well as intestinally digestible forms. Studies in which up to 5 g/day was used reported increased growth of hair fibre in goats (Souri *et al.*, 1998; Galbraith *et al.*, 1998) and rates of growth of wall horn in goats (Galbraith *et al.*, 1998) and dairy cows (15 g/day) (Metcalf *et al.*, 1998).

Table 1. Relative composition of selected amino acids (g amino acid/16 g N) in tissues and dietary protein sources. After Galbraith and Scaife (2008).

Amino acid	Wall horn	Sole horn	Muscle	Rumen microbial protein	Extracted soyabean meal	White fishmeal
Threonine	5.2	4.8	3.9	5.2	4.2	4.2
Leucine	8.1	8.9	5.8	7.4	8.2	6.7
Phenylalanine	2.3	1.4	3.1	5.5	5.5	3.9
Lysine	5.1	1.4	5.9	8.1	6.8	5.7
Methionine	0.70	1.04	1.8	2.5	1.4	3.0
Cyst(e)ine	6.51	4.05	1.1	1.0	1.4	0.9

A marked increase in the growth rate of the hoof horn *post partum* and resistance to wear was observed in primiparous lactating Holstein heifers supplemented with methionine (Livesey and Laven, 2007). The addition of rumen-protected L-methionine (5-6 g/day) to the feed of dairy heifers throughout pregnancy increased methionine blood concentrations (23.2 vs 19.2 µmol/l) but had no impact on growth characteristics and concentrations of L-methionine or L-cysteine in claw wall horn collected 2-3 days post partum (Galbraith *et al.*, 2006). In contrast, Clark and Rakes (1982) reported an increase in growth rates and reduction in the concentration of cysteine in upper wall claw horn of dairy cattle supplemented with 30 g/day of methionine hydroxy analogue for 70-90 days.

In a recent study using bovine hoof explants Hepburn *et al.* (2008) used ^{35}S-methionine to measure the rate of L-methionine uptake, its rate of incorporation into protein and its effects on the stimulation of DNA synthesis. Uptake reached steady state conditions within 30 minutes at which time K_m and V_{max} were 3.61 mmol/litre and 5.84 mmol/kg intracellular water/30 min, respectively. Uptake of L-methionine was not influenced by L-cysteine or L-cystine. Maximum rates of methionine incorporation into protein occurred at a methionine concentration of approximately 50 mmol/l, which is within the physiological range for methionine concentration. Hepburn *et al.* (2008) suggested that maximization of proliferative and protein depositional activity in solear epidermis and dermis *in vivo* would require the delivery of systemic concentrations of 50 mmol/l L-methionine.

5.2. Lipids

In the bovine claw lipids have a functional significance as an important part of the cementing substance between differentiating epidermal cells of the horn and in the digital cushions located below the pedal bone. In the former, the nature of the lipids and the long chain fatty acids they contain, suggests very specialised *in situ* lipogenesis. Lipids in the bovine horn tissue were first described by Ueta *et al.* (1971) as containing cholesterol (31%), free fatty acids (24%), triacylglycerols (10%), cholesterol sulphate (7%), and sphingolipids (16%). The total lipid content of hoof horn is low with values of 1.5% for wall horn and 3% for sole horn and is characterised by the presence of very long chain fatty acids (>C24) (Table 2) (Scaife *et al.*, 2000). Similarly, Hamanaka *et al.* (2002) reported that the sphingolipid fraction of epidermal lipids, which consisted predominantly of ceramides and glucosylceramides, contained very long chain α- and ω-hydroxylated fatty acids. In skin, which contains a

Table 2. Fatty acid composition of bovine non-hydroxy fatty acids (g/kg total fatty acids). Taken from Scaife et al. *(2000).*

Fatty acid	Sole	Heel	Wall
C16:0	21.4	26.5	26.2
C16:1	6.3	4.1	1.5
C18:0	8.3	11.0	1.3
C18:1	10.8	10.0	13.4
C18:2	11.9	8.2	9.7
C18:3	3.3	2.7	5.9
C20-24	13.9	11.9	1.3
>C24	8.5	7.5	8.3

similar lipid and fatty acid profile, these long chain fatty acid-containing lipids have been likened to 'molecular rivets' providing adhesion between adjacent cornified epidermal cells (Wertz and Downing, 1991). There is some evidence that the fatty acid composition of hoof horn can be influenced by dietary fatty acids and that polyunsaturated fatty acids of marine origin can be incorporated into the horn lipid fraction (Offer and Logue, 1998; Offer *et al.*, 2000).

Of particular interest is the role of lipids in the digital cushions, which act as shock absorbers between the pedal bone and the soft tissues of the sole. Evidence suggests the lipid is predominantly triacylglycerol containing a fatty acid composition similar to that in the diet and, therefore, susceptible to dietary manipulation. Changes in the physical characteristics of these digital cushions may change the protection they afford the underlying dermal and epidermal tissues from the stresses placed upon them by the pedal bone and the likelihood of lesions forming. There is little detailed information on the fatty acid composition of the lipids in the digital cushions although Raber *et al.* (2004) and (2006) have recently reported preliminary data on the lipid content and fatty acid composition of the digital cushions from Brown Swiss heifers and cows fed a maize silage, grass and hay diet. The mean lipid content of the digital cushions was significantly lower in heifers (264 g/kg tissue) compared with cows (367 g/kg tissue) and was markedly lower than typical values of 870-940 g/kg tissue for the total fatty acid content of perinephric adipose tissue depots in the same animals. There were major differences in the lipid content of the six different fat pads isolated from each claw (74-431 g/kg tissue in heifers and 133-619 g/kg tissue in cows). Anatomically, two of the cushions which contained the lowest fat content were located in the region of the claw where sole ulcers are likely to develop. This observation suggested that there was inadequate cushioning to prevent impact damage to underlying soft tissue. The fatty acid content of the digital cushion was shown not to be typical of subcutaneous and perinephric adipose tissue in containing a higher proportion of monounsaturated fatty acids, predominantly $C18:1n-9$, and lower proportions of saturated fatty acids. These data suggest tissue-specific synthesis of fatty acids or modification of absorbed fatty acids by desaturation to achieve the elevated MUFA content. This may be important to ensure that the digital cushions have the appropriate physical characteristics, which enable them to deform under load.

To date there is no information on the way in which the fat content or fatty acid composition of the digital cushions responds to nutritional influences and physiological state. Previous studies in non-ruminants have shown that dietary fatty acids can markedly influence the fatty acid composition of adipose tissue (Onibi *et al.*, 2000; Scaife *et al.*, 1994) and in ruminants the feeding of rumen protected lipids can achieve similar changes in the composition of adipose tissue depots (Scollan *et al.*, 2003). It is important to understand the factors, which influence the content and composition of fatty acids in the digital cushions in order to better manage cow nutrition. If the mobilisation of fat from adipose tissues depots in early lactation cows (Bauman and Currie, 1980) also occurs in the digital cushions, this may have important consequences for the development lameness. The advent of functional foods and the greater interest in manipulation milk fatty acid composition through the targeted use of rumen protected fatty acids supplements (Jenkins and McGuire, 2006) may also have consequences for the functionality of the digital cushions and the occurrence of lameness.

5.3. Vitamins and minerals

The formation of hoof horn is a complex process involving a number of different tissues and vitamins and minerals are recognised to have an important influence on events. Vitamins considered important because of their roles in keratinisation and cell differentiation, calcium homeostasis, and cellular antioxidant protection, respectively are biotin and vitamins A, D and E. Of the vitamins, biotin has received most attention. Very few studies have investigated the effect of biotin deficiency in cattle, however, in non-ruminant species it has long been known that disorders in skin and other integumental tissue, including hoof horn are associated with induced or naturally occurring deficiency and respond to dietary biotin supplementation. Several studies have now demonstrated that daily dietary biotin supplementation (typically 20 mg/day) can improve claw integrity and reduce lameness. In a recent review, Green and Mülling (2005) summarised a number of field studies designed to investigate the effect of long term biotin supplementation in the incidence of claw lesions. Studies in Australia (Fitzgerald *et al.*, 2000), Europe (Distl and Schmid, 1994; Hagemeister and Steinberg, 1996; Hedges *et al.*, 2001 and Bergsten *et al.*, 2004) and Canada (Campbell *et al.*, 2000) support the view that locomotion score is improved and the incidence of lameness, sole ulcers, heel erosion, vertical fissures and sand cracks reduced by long term oral biotin supplementation, typically 12 to 18 months, at a dose rate of 10-20 mg biotin per day.

Biotin supplementation appears to be most effective in reducing white line disease. The white line is often considered a mechanically weak area of the claw because it is composed of heterogenous horn different in their sites of production, i.e. the wall and sole. Morphological and biochemical studies suggest that biotin improves the properties of the intercellular cementing substance between epidermal cells and thus can increase the strength of the white line (Budras *et al.*, 1996). In summarising papers by Midla *et al.* (1998), Hedges *et al.* (2001), Hoblet *et al.* (2002) and Potzsch *et al.* (2003), Green and Mulling (2005) concluded that epidemiological evidence supports the view that daily supplementation with 20mg biotin for 6 months resulted in a reduction in lameness and foot lesions. The mechanisms by which biotin brings about this reduction in lameness are poorly understood. In addition to its well established roles in lipid metabolism, amino acid metabolism, cellular respiration and gluconeogenesis, it has recently been shown to have a number of non-carboxylase functions, which may, in part, explain its effects in claw horn. These functions, which include regulation of gene expression, biotinylation of histones and effects on cellular proliferation have recently been reviewed by Zempleni (2005).

The benefits of biotin supplementation suggest that in modern dairy cows the production of biotin in the rumen is insufficient to meet the needs to the animal. There is remarkably little information on ruminal production of biotin and the influence of diet. The proportion of free biotin (water soluble biotin) present in feedstuffs can vary from 10 to 80% of the total biotin present. In general the proportion of free biotin is higher in feedstuffs of plant origin compared with those of animal origin. The 'free' biotin fraction may also contain biocytin in which biotin is linked to lysine. A number of the microbiological assays used to estimate free biotin also measure biotin bound in biocytin (Bonjour, 1991).

NRC (1978) recommends 10 mg biotin/kg body weight for dairy calves and indicates that microbial synthesis of biotin is adequate for adult dairy cattle. NRC (2001) makes no specific recommendation for biotin on the basis that the available scientific data is inadequate. The limited evidence available from *in vitro* and *in vivo* studies suggests that diet has a significant effect on the synthesis and/or degradation of microbial and dietary biotin. Studies *in vitro*, using a RUSITEC system suggest that forage-based diets favour microbial biotin synthesis and that as the proportion of concentrate in the diet increases the rumen biotin balance is markedly reduced (Table 3). In a study in duodenally cannulated dairy cows, Lebzien *et al.* (2006) reported that the duodenal flow of biotin was not related to biotin intake but to the amount of fermentable organic matter and microbial protein. In their study ruminal biotin balance was positive for diets containing a mixture of forage and concentrate and negative for a hay only diet.

Evidence for beneficial effects of supplementation with vitamins other than biotin is less clear although a biochemical rationale can be argued for a number of candidate vitamins. Vitamin A is known to be an important regulator of cell differentiation and its deficiency is associated with abnormalities in epithelial tissues, often associated with an increase in cellular keratinisation. The link with vitamin A is thought to be through its influence on gene expression in epithelial cells (Tomlinson *et al.*, 2004). Vitamin D may impact on the differentiation of the epidermal layers of the hoof through its influence on calcium availability. Some recent *in vitro* data suggest that differentiating epidermal cells are particularly sensitive to fluctuations in calcium concentration (Micallef *et*

Table 3. Influence of forage:concentrate ratio on biotin balance in a RUSITEC system (adapted from Abel et al., 2001).

Feed (g/d) Hay + barley	Biotin (µg/d)			
	Feed	Solid digesta	Liquid phase	Balance
10+2	2.49[e]	0.88[b]	3.14[b]	1.53[b]
6+6	2.27[c]	0.62[a]	2.42[ab]	0.77[ab]
2+10	2.02[a]	0.47[a]	1.89[a]	0.34[a]

Mean values with different superscripts are significantly different ($P<0.05$).
Balance = biotin in feed – (biotin in solid digesta and liquid phase).

al., 2008). Vitamin E may provide antioxidant protection to unsaturated fatty acids in the lipids of the digital cushion and intercellular cementing substance but there is no direct evidence to suggest direct beneficial effects of vitamin E supplementation on hoof health. More likely, its effects will be seen through its involvement in the immune response, most probably by protecting neutrophils against damage caused by free radicals generated during phagocytosis (Kilic *et al.*, 2007) of bacteria present at the site of hoof lesions.

Tomlinson *et al.* (2004) identified calcium, zinc, copper, selenium and manganese as minerals required for keratinisation during hoof formation and Wilde (2006) and Andrieu (2008) have reviewed the role of macro- and micro-minerals in the dairy cow. Studies *in vitro* have demonstrated that differentiating epidermal cells are very sensitive to changes in calcium concentration (Micallef *et al.*, 2008). Such changes, which are likely to occur at the time of parturition and onset of lactation, have the potential to influence the metabolism and differentiation of epidermal cells. In addition, epidermal transglutaminase is required to cross-link keratin fibres during the keratinisation process in horn epidermis. An insufficiency in local calcium due to inadequate dietary supply, poor absorption (perhaps related to vitamin D status) and excretion of calcium in milk may lead to the formation of dyskeratotic horn (Tomlinson *et al.*, 2004).

It has been suggested that zinc has three key roles in the keratinisation process. These are catalytic roles carried out by Zn metalloenzymes, structural roles in zinc finger proteins and regulatory roles through its effects on calmodulin, protein kinase C, thyroid binding hormone and inositol phosphate synthesis. Copper is a cofactor in thiol oxidase, which is involved in the formation of disulphide bridges between cysteine residues in keratin. This process is essential for structural strength of the keratinised cell matrix of hoof horn. In a recent study to compare supply of Zn, Mn, Cu and Co as complexed trace minerals with supply in the inorganic form, Nocek *et al.* (2006) concluded that the reproductive and health performance of cows provided with the NRC (2001) requirements for these minerals in the complexed form was similar to cows provided with the same mineral in the inorganic form. However, white line separation was lower in animals given the complexed minerals. Enjalbert *et al.* (2006) conducted a retrospective study of French and Belgian dairy and beef herds to examine the relationship between trace element status and health and performance. Herds studied were categorised as deficient, marginal, low-adequate or high-adequate for copper, zinc and selenium based on blood parameters. The study indicated a relationship between zinc deficiency and impaired locomotion, which is in accord with previous studies that have shown lameness and hoof deformation in zinc deficient animals (Lamand and Perigaud, 1973; Corbellini *et al.*, 1997) and improved hoof quality scores in beef cattle supplemented with 10 mg zinc/kg DM supplied as a protein complex (Bioplex) or as a polysaccharide complex (Kessler *et al.*, 2003).

Selenium is required for naturally occurring selenoproteins in the hoof, among these is glutathione peroxidise which contributes to the antioxidant protection mechanisms of hoof tissue. (Tomlinson *et al.*, 2004). Claw horn disorders are associated with toxic levels of dietary selenium usually as a result of prolonged or excessive consumption of seleniferous plants (O'Toole and Raisbeck, 1995). In these rare situations excess selenium (i.e. that not incorporated at specific sites into naturally occurring selenoproteins) may accumulate as the selenoamino acids, selenocysteine and selonomethionine. There is evidence that these selenoamino acids are used to replace, unspecifically, sulphur-containing amino acids in the synthesis of a number of animal proteins and it is likely that they are incorporated into keratins and associated proteins. Current information suggests that unspecific incorporation of selenomethionine into protein is relatively well tolerated (Schrauzer, 2000) but similar assimilation of selenocysteine may lead to toxicity and potential interference with, for example, the formation of disulphide bridges required for keratinisation and synthesis of good quality horn (Tomlinson *et al.*, 2004). This explanation would be consistent with the observations that excess dietary selenium intake has a major impact on the integrity of hoof horn keratin and leads to lesion development (O'Toole and Raisbeck, 1995).

6. Conclusions

The bovine claw is a complex structure, the function of which is influenced by environmental, physiological and nutritional factors. The good management of dairy cow nutrition from birth to the end of their productive life can influence the incidence of lameness and has the potential to prolong the productive period. The tissues in the claw are sensitive to the quantity and quality of nutrient supply. The avascular nature of the hoof epidermal tissues means that metabolic activity and the synthesis of good quality horn are dependent on blood flow to the dermis to deliver nutrients, which are destined to be either structural components of the hoof tissues or which have a metabolic and regulatory role. Fluctuations in either blood flow or nutrient availability can have a detrimental effect on structure and functionality of the hoof and good feeding management and ration formulation can minimise the likelihood of acidosis and ensure the adequate supply of individual nutrients to the hoof. The consequences of lameness are pain and suffering for the animal and reduced reproductive and lactational performance affecting economic returns for the producer. With the continuing drive towards greater productivity from individual animals, lameness is likely to remain a serious issue. However, its impact may be reduced by a better understanding of the role of nutrients in maintaining claw health and in the application of this knowledge in good nutritional practice.

References

Abel, H.J., I. Immig, C. Da Costa Gomez and W. Steinberg, 2001. Research note: Effect of increasing dietary concentrate level on microbial biotin metabolism in the artificial rumen simulation system (RUSITEC). *Archives of Animal Nutrition* 55:371-376.

Andrieu, S., 2008. Is there a role for organic trace element supplements in transition cow health? *Veterinary Record* **176**:77-83.

Bauman, D.E. and W.B. Currie, 1980. Partitioning of nutrients during pregnancy and lactation: A review of mechanisms involving homeostasis and homeorhesis. *Journal of Dairy Science* **63**:1514-1529.

Bergsten, C., P.R. Greenough. J.M. Gay, W.M. Seymour and C.C. Gay, 2004. Effects of biotin supplementation on performance and claw lesions on a commercial dairy farm. *Journal of Dairy Science* **86**:3953-3962.

Bonjour, J-P., 1991. Biotin. In: *Handbook of Vitamins*, L. Machlin (Ed.) J. Dekker, New York, USA, pp. 393-427.

Budras, K.-D. and A. Wünsche, 2002. *Atlas der Anatomie des Rindes*. Schlütersche GmBH & Co., Hannover, Germany.

Budras, K.D., H. Geyer, J. Maierl and C.K.W. Mülling, 1998. Anatomy and structure of hoof horn (Workshop report). In: *10th International Symposium on Lameness in Ruminants*, C.J. Lischer and P. Ossent (Eds.) University of Zurich, Switzerland, pp. 176-199.

Budras, K.D., C. Mülling and A. Horowitz, 1996. The rate of keratinisation of the wall segment of the cattle hoof and its relationship to width and structure of the zona alba (white line) with respect to claw disease. *American Journal of Veterinary Research* 57:444-455.

Campbell, J., P.R. Greenough and L. Petrie, 2000. The effect of biotin on sandcracks in beef cattle. *Canadian Veterinary Journal* **41**:690-694.

Clark, A.K. and A.H. Rakes, 1982. Effect of methionine hydroxy analog supplementation on dairy cattle hoof growth and composition. *Journal of Dairy Science* **65**:1493-1502.

Corbellini, C.N., A.R. Mangoni, A.C. De Mattos and J. Auzmendi, 1997. Effects of supplementation of slightly deficient dairy cows with zinc oxide or methionine zinc. *Revista de Medicinia Veterinaria* **78**:439-447.

Distl, O. and D. Schmid, 1994. The influence of biotin supplementation on the conformation,hardness and health of claws of dairy cows. *Tierärztliche Umschau* **49**:581-584.

Enjalert, F., P. Lebreton and O. Salat, 2006. Effects of copper, zinc and selenium status on performance and health in commercial dairy and beef herds: retrospective study. *Journal of Animal Physiology and Nutrition* **90**:459-466.

Fitzgerald, T., B.W. Norton, R. Elliott and O. Svendsen, 2000. The influence of long-term supplementation with biotin on the prevention of lameness in pasture fed dairy cows. *Journal of Dairy Science* **83**:338-344.

Galbraith, H., 1995. The effects of diet on nutrient partition in Scottish Cashmere and Angora goats. In: *The nutrition and grazing ecology of speciality fibre animals*, J.P. Laker, and A.J.F. Russel (Eds.) European Fine Fibre Network Publication No. 3. Macaulay land Use Research Institutte, Aberdeen, UK, pp. 23-50.

Galbraith, H., H. Rae, T. Omand, K.A.K. Hendry, C.H. Knight and C.J. Wilde, 2006. Effect of supplementing pregnant heifers with methionine or melatonin on the anatomy and other characteristics of their lateral hind claws. *Veterinary Record* **156**:21-24.

Galbraith, H., M. Mengal and J.R. Scaife, 1998. Effect of dietary methionine and biotin supplementation on growth and protein and amino acid composition of caprine hoof horn. In: *10th International Symposium on Lameness in Ruminants*, Ch.J. Lischer and P. Ossent (Eds.). Lucerne, Switzerland, pp. 227-229.

Galbraith, H and J.R. Scaife, 2008. Lameness in dairy cows: Influence of nutrition on claw composition and health In: *Recent advances in animal nutrition 2007*, Garnsworthy and Wiseman (Eds.), Nottingham University Press, UK, pp. 61-97.

Green, L. and C.K.W. Muelling, 2005. Biotin and lameness – a review. *Cattle Practice* **13**:145-153.

Greenough, P.R., A.D. Weaver, D.M. Broom, R.J. Esslemont and F.A. Galindo, 1997. Basic concepts of lameness. In: *Lameness in cattle*, P.R. Greenough and A.D. Weaver (Eds.), W.B Saunders Company, Philadelphia, USA, pp. 3-13.

Hagemeister, H. and W. Steinberg, 1996. Effects of a long-term dietary biotin administration on claw health in dairy cows. In: *Proceeding of 9th International Symposium on Disorders in the Bovine Digit*, Jerusalem, Israel.

Hamanaka S., M. Hara, H. Nishio, F. Otsuka, S. Suzuki and Y. Uchida, 2002. Human epidermal glucosylceramides are major precursors of stratum corneum ceramides. *Journal of Investigative Dermatology* **119**:416-23.

Hedges, J., R.W. Blowey, A.J. Packington, C.J. O'Callaghan and L.E. Green, 2001. A longitudinal field trial of the effect of biotin supplementation on lameness in dairy cows. *Journal of Dairy Science* **84**:1969-1975.

Hepburn, N.L., C.H. Knight, C.J. Wilde, K.A.K. Hendry and H. Galbraith, 2008. Methionine uptake, incorporation and effects on proliferative activity and protein synthesis in bovine claw tissue explants in vitro. *Journal of Agricultural Science* **146**:103-115.

Hoblet, K., W. Weiss, D. Anderson and M. Moeschberger, 2002. Effect of oral biotin supplementation. In: *Proceedings of 12th International Symposium on Lameness in Ruminants*, J.K., Shearer (Ed.) Orlando, USA, pp. 253-255.

Jenkins, T.C. and M.A. McGuire, 2006. Major advances in nutrition: impact on milk composition. *Journal of Dairy Science* **89**:1302-1310.

Kessler, J., I. Moreol, P-A. Dufey, A. Gutzwiller, A. Stern and H. Geyer, 2003. Efect of organic zinc sources on performance, zinc status and carcass, meat and claw quality in fattening bulls. *Livestock Production Science* **81**:161-171.

Keunen, J.E., J.C. Plaizier, L. Kyriasakis, T.F. Duffield, T.M. Widowski, M.I. Lindinger and B.W. McBride, 2002. Effects of a subacute acidosis model on the diet selection of dairy cows. *Journal of Dairy Science* **85**:3304-3313.

Kilic, N., A. Ceylan, I. Serin and C. Gokbulut, 2007. Possible interaction between lameness, fertility, some minerals and vitamin E in dairy cows. *Bulletin of Veterinary Institute Pulawy* **51**:425-429.

Lamand, M. and S. Perigaud, 1973. Carences en oligo-éléments en France. 1. Eléments d'enquête obtenus dans la pratique vétéinaire. *Annales de Recherches Veterinaires* **4**:513-534.

Leach, K.A., J.E. Offer, I. Svoboda and D.N. Logue, 2005. Effects of type of forage fed to dairy heifers: Associations between claw characteristics, clinical lameness, environment and behaviour. *Veterinary Journal* **169**:427-436.

Lebzien, P., H. Abel, B. Schröder and G. Flachowsky, 2006. Studies on the biotin flow at the duodenum of dairy cows fed diets with different concentrate levels and types of forages. *Archives of Animal Nutrition* **60**:80-88.

Livesey, C.T. and R.A. Laven, 2007. Effects of housing and intake of methionine on the growth and wear of hoof horn and the conformation of the hooves of first-lactation Holstein heifers. *Veterinary Record* **160**:470-476.

Lischer, C.J. and P. Ossent, 2000. Sole ulcers in dairy cattle – What's new about an old disease. In: *11th Symposium on Disorders of the Ruminant Digit*, C.M. Mortellaro, L. De Vecchis and A. Brizzi (Eds.) Parma, Italy, pp. 46-55.

Logue, D.N., J.E. Offer and S.A. Kempson, 1993. Lameness in dairy cattle. *Irish Veterinary Journal* **46**:47-58.

Metcalf, J.A., C. Marsh, A.M. Johnston, S.A. May and C.T. Livesey, 1998. Effect of dietary methionine supplementation on hoof horn growth in primiparous cows. In: *Proceedings of the British Society of Animal Science*, Penicuik, p. 200.

Micallef, L., F. Belaubre, A. Pinon, C. Jayat-Vignoles, C. Delage, M. Charveron and A. Simon, 2008. Effects of extracellular calcium on the growth-differentiation switch in immortalized keratinocyte HaCaT cells compared with normal human keratinocytes. *Experimental Dermatology*, Epub ahead of print.

Midla, L.T., K.H. Hoblet, W.P. Weiss and M.L. Moescheberger, 1998. Supplemental dietary biotin for prevention of lesions associated with aseptic subclinical laminitis (*pododermatitis aseptical diffusa*) in primiparous cows. *American Journal of Veterinary Research* **59**:733-738.

Mülling, C.K.W., R.Y. Wustenberg, U. Nebel, D. Hoffmann and K.D. Budras, 2006. Innovative *in vitro* and *ex vivo* models in multidisciplinary european lameness research. *Cattle Practice* **14**:115-122.

Nocek, J.E., M.T. Socha and D.J. Tomlinson, 2006. The effect of trace mineral fortification level and source on performance of dairy cattle. *Journal of Dairy Science* **89**:2679-2693.

NRC, 1978. *Nutrient requirements for domestic animals. No 3. Nutrient requirements of dairy cows*, 5th Ed., National Academy of Sciences. National Research Council, Washington, DC.

NRC, 2001. *Nutrient requirements of dairy cows*, 7th Rev. Ed., National Academic Press, Washington, DC., pp. 162-177.

Offer, J.E. and D.N. Logue, 1998. The effect of lameness in the dairy cow on the fatty acid profile of claw horn lipids. In: *Proceedings of the 10th International Symposium on Ruminant Lameness*, C.J. Lischer and P. Ossent (Eds.) University of Zurich, Switzerland, pp. 220-221.

Offer, J.E., N.W. Offer and D.N. Logue, 2000. Effects of dietary fish oil supplementation on the hoof lipid fatty acid profiles of dairy cattle. In: *Proceedings of the XI International Symposium on Disorders of the Ruminant Digit*, C.M. Mortellaro, L. De Veechis and A. Brizzi (eds.). Parma, Italy, pp. 322-324.

Offer, J.E., K.A. Leach, S. Brocklehurst and D.N. Logue, 2003. Effect of forage type on claw horn lesion development in dairy heifers. *Veterinary Journal* **165**:221-227.

Onibi, G.E., J.R. Scaife, I. Murray and V.R. Fowler, 2000. Supplementary a-tocopherol acetate in full-fat rapeseed-based diets for pigs: influence on tissue a-tocopherol content, fatty acid profiles and lipid oxidation. *Journal of the Science of Food and Agriculture* **80**:1625-1632.

O'Toole, D. and M.F. Raisbeck, 1995. Pathology of experimentally induced chronic selenosis (alkali disease) in yearling cattle. *Journal of Veterinary Diagnostic Investigation* **7**:364-373.

Owens, F.N., D.S. Secrist, W.J. Hill. and D.R. Gill, 1998. Acidosis in cattle: a review. *Journal of Animal Science* **76**:275-286.

Potzsch, C.J., V.J. Collis, R.W. Blowey, A.J. Packington and L.E. Green, 2003. The impact of parity and duration of biotin supplementation on white line disease lameness in dairy cattle. *Journal of Dairy Science* **86**:2577-2582.

Raber, M., C.J. Lischer, H. Geyer and P. Ossent, 2004. The bovine digital cushion – a descriptive anatomical study. *Veterinary Journal* **176**:258-264.

Raber, M., M.R.L. Scheeder, P. Ossent, C.J. Lischer and H. Geyer, 2006. The content and composition of lipids in the digital cushion of the bovine claw with respect to age and location-a preliminary report. *Veterinary Journal* **172**:173-177.

Reis, P.J., 1989. The influence of absorbed nutrients on wool growth. In: *The biology of wool and hair*, G.E. Rogers, P.J. Reis, K.A. Ward and R.C. Marshall (Eds.). Chapman and Hall, Cambridge, UK, pp. 185-204.

Scaife, J.R., J. Moyo, H. Galbraith, W. Michie and V. Campbell, 1994. Effect of different dietary supplemental fats and oils on the growth performance and tissue fatty acid composition of female broilers. *British Poultry Science* **35**:107-118.

Scaife, J., K. Meyer and E. Grant, 2000. Comparison of the lipids of the bovine and equine hoof horn. In: *Proceedings of the XI International Symposium on Disorders of the Runinant Digit*, C.M. Mortellaro, L. De Veechis and A. Brizzi (Eds.). Parma, Italy, pp. 125-127.

Schrauzer, G.N., 2000. Selenomethionine: a review of its nutritional significance, metabolism and toxicity. *Journal of Nutrition* **130**:1653-1656.

Scollan N.D., M. Enser, S.K. Gulati, I. Richardson and J.D. Wood, 2003. Effects of including a ruminally protected lipid supplement in the diet on the fatty acid composition of beef muscle. *British Journal of Nutrition* **90**:709-716.

Souri, M., H. Galbraith and J.R. Scaife, 1998. Comparisons of the effect of protected methionine supplementation on growth, digestive characteristics and fibre yield in Cashmere-yielding and Angora goats. *Animal Science* **66**:217-223.

Stone, W.C., 2004. Nutritional approaches to minimize subacute ruminal acidosis and laminitis in dairy cattle. *Journal of Dairy Science* **87**:E13-E26.

Tarlton, J.F., D.E. Holah, K.M. Evans, S. Jones, G.R. Pearson and A.J.F. Webster, 2003. Biomechanical and histological changes in the support structures of bovine hooves around the time of first calving. *Veterinary Journal* **162**:56-65.

Tomlinson, D.J., C.H. Muelling and T.M. Fakler, 2004. Formation of keratins in the bovine claw: roles of hormones, minerals and vitamins in functional claw integrity. *Journal of Dairy Science* **87**:797-809.

Ueta, N., S. Kawamura, I. Kanazawa and T. Yamakawa, 1971. On the nature of so-called ungulic acid. *Journal of Biochemistry* **70**:881-883.

Van Amstel, S.R., J.K. Shearer and F.L. Palin, 2004. Moisture content, thickness and lesions of sole horn associated with thin soles in dairy cattle. *Journal of Dairy Science* **87**:757-763.

Vermunt, J.J., 2004. Herd lameness-a review, major causal factors and guidelines for prevention and control. In: *13th International Symposium on Lameness in ruminants*, B. Zemljic (ed.), Maribor, pp. 3-18.

Webster, A.J.F., L. Knott and J.F. Tarlton, 2005. Understanding lameness in the dairy cow. *Cattle Practice* **13**:93-98.

Wertz, P.W. and D.T. Downing, 1991. Epidermal lipids. In: *Physiology, biochemistry and molecular biology of the skin*, 2nd Edition, L.A. Goldsmith (Ed.) Oxford University Press, New York, USA, pp. 205-236.

Wilde, D., 2006. Influence of macro and micro minerals in the peri-parturient period on fertility in dairy cattle. *Animal Reproduction Science* **96**:240-249.

Zemplini, J., 2005. Uptake, location and noncarboxylase roles of biotin. *Annual Reviews of Nutrition* **25**:175-196.

Role of mycotoxins in cow health and immunity

R.R. Santos and J. Fink-Gremmels
Division Veterinary Pharmacology, Pharmacy and Toxicology, Faculty of Veterinary Medicine, Utrecht University, Utrecht, the Netherlands

1. Introduction

In an ecological balance, plants and moulds (*fungi imperfecti*) are in mutual symbiosis. Symbiotic moulds produce a number of secondary metabolites that protect plants and their seeds against bacteria and parasites, and improve the resistance of plants to environmental stress factors (Schardl *et al.*, 1996; Fink-Gremmels, 2005). However, several of these fungal metabolites are toxic to animals and humans. These metabolites are referred to as mycotoxins. Related fungal metabolites may have beneficial effects for the plant and may also be useful in the therapy of certain diseases in humans and animals. The most well-known example of beneficial substances is the penicillins, which are widely used as antibiotics in veterinary and human therapy, and which originate from *Penicillium* species.

Contamination of food and feed commodities with one or more hazardous mycotoxins is of global concern. Food safety measures address particularly those toxins that are proven or suspected carcinogens, such as aflatoxins, ochratoxins and fumonisins. Their occurrence in foods and feeds is regularly measured to avoid or reduce the rate of contamination and a format for reporting these findings has been established in Europe. For other toxins, reporting is often not standardised, although these are found with a high prevalence in Europe. This applies for the group of trichothecenes but also for many *Penicillium* toxins.

In animal feeds, mycotoxin contamination can be a consequence of pre- and post-harvest invasion by multiple fungal species. These fungal species often produce more than one toxin and different fungi can invade the same feed material prior to harvest or during storage. This complex exposure pattern makes it difficult to evaluate and quantify the detrimental effects of mycotoxins under practical conditions. It is generally assumed that monogastric species, such as pigs and poultry are amongst the most sensitive animals species, whereas ruminants are less susceptible. The latter is attributed to the natural barrier formed by the rumen and its microbiological flora. Rumen microorganisms are able to degrade and inactivate many mycotoxins, preventing systemic exposure of the animal and the occurrence of adverse reactions. However, several mycotoxins, such as fumonisins and ergot alkaloids, pass the rumen flora without being metabolised, and are absorbed from the intestines in their biologically active form. Moreover, a dysfunction of the rumen flora and long-term exposure might decrease the capacity of the rumen microorganisms to inactivate mycotoxins. In all these cases intact mycotoxins will reach the systemic circulation and produce signs of intoxication comparable to those seen in monogastric species.

It is the aim of this brief review to illustrate how dairy cows can be exposed to mycotoxins and what consequences this exposure might have on animal health and immunity.

2. Mycotoxins in the diet of dairy cows

The potential sources of mycotoxins in the diet of dairy cows are the concentrates, silages and forage grasses. Diet composition may vary significantly between geographic regions, reflecting extensive animal husbandry where the diet consists mainly of pasture grass and an intensive production in feedlots or high-producing farms, where the major part of the diet is given in the form of a concentrate. Animal performance depends on the intake of digestible and metabolisable nutrients, and the optimal composition of a diet in the different production stages of a dairy cow is a matter of ongoing research in the area of animal nutrition. Regarding mycotoxin exposure, three major sources need to be discussed: (a) grains, maize (corn) and other protein-rich commodities as present in concentrates, (b) fresh forages and (c) preserved forages, such as silages and haylage (wrapped bales).

2.1. Mycotoxins in concentrates

Grains and maize are susceptible to *Fusarium* species that invade the living plant. Toxin production occurs at the pre-harvest stage, and comprises the large group of trichothecenes with more than 180 individual toxins, of which deoxynivalenol (DON), nivalenol (NIV), diatoxyscirpenol (DAS) and their derivatives are the most commonly investigated and measured toxins. Maize and products thereof are frequently contaminated with zearalenone and fumonisins, which are produced by the same *Fusarium* species (as for example *F. graminearum*, which produces trichothecenes, as well as zearalenone) or by specialist fungi, such as *F. verticilloides*, the most prominent producer of fumonisins.

An entirely different group of mycotoxins are the alkaloids. Main producers are *Claviceps* species, which are now allocated to the group of endophytes. Endophytes are the predominant fungal species in fresh forage grasses (see following section), but some *Claviceps* species also invade small grains resulting in a contamination with ergot alkaloids.

Aflatoxins occur in many energy-rich concentrates as, for example, cereal grains, maize gluten, soybean products, as well as in press cakes from oil plants, such as peanuts, sunflower seeds, cotton seeds, palm kernels, and coprah. Contamination with aflatoxin-producing *Aspergilli* is assumed to take place particularly at the post-harvest stage during storage, but pre-harvest contamination has been demonstrated as well. The same applies for the ochratoxins, common mycotoxins in small grains.

This very brief and far from complete overview illustrates the diversity of mycotoxins that can be present in concentrates. Due to the entirely different structure of the individual mycotoxins, no general calculation of the total mycotoxin burden of the animal can be made. As mentioned already in the introduction, the rumen flora metabolises trichothecenes and zearalenone, as well as aflatoxins and ochratoxins, whereas many ergot alkaloids and the fumonisins pass through the rumen and reach the small intestine in their biologically active form (for details on rumen metabolism of the individual mycotoxins see Jouany and Diaz, 2005). Hence the internal dose of a toxin, i.e. the amount that is absorbed in the small intestine needs to be calculated for each individual toxin.

2.2. Mycotoxins in fresh forages

Pasture grasses (forages) are particularly at risk from invasion by endophytes. Endophytes are characterised by a typical life cycle describing whether or not fungal infection between plants is seed transmitted or dependent on vectors, such as plant eating flies. Endophytes are one of the most perfect examples for a valuable symbiosis of plants and fungal species, as they convey stress resistance and resistance to many plant parasites. Toxins produced by these endophytes comprise the group of ergot alkaloids. The contamination of Tall fescue, the major forage grass in central and south-eastern United States, with ergovaline and related ergot alkaloids accounts for example for significant economic losses among cattle farmers each year. Another group of toxins belongs to the chemical class of indole-derivatives, of which lolitrem B is the most prominent representative occurring on perennial ryegrass. Initially reports on intoxications involving lolitrem B were only reported in Australia and New Zealand, but in the last decennia, toxin-producing *Neothyphodium* species have been found on all continents and the level of contamination of cold season grasses is of increasing concern (for review see Fink-Gremmels, 2005).

2.3. Mycotoxins in preserved forages

A common observation at the farm level is the occurrence of moulds in stored or ensiled feeds. In silages, a variety of mould species can be detected including *Penicillium* spp., *Byssochlamus* spp., *Aspergillus fumigatus* and *Trichoderma* spp. These fungal species have gained less attention regarding their ability to produce mycotoxins and have been primarily addressed as spoilage moulds, accounting for a loss of structure, and an adverse (mouldy) taste of the silage. This adverse taste is well recognised by dairy cows and associated with a reduced feed intake. However, laboratory and field studies showed that these mould species produce a variety of toxins in silage, the most prominent ones being patulin, as well as mycophenolic acid and the roquefortins. In a recent study, Mansfield *et al.* (2008) have demonstrated the presence of four *Penicillium* mycotoxins (patulin, mycophenolic acid, cyclopiazonic acid and roquefortine C) in fresh and ensiled maize, contradicting the belief that toxin formation occurs exclusively during storage. The final concentration of these mycotoxins can be affected by climate conditions prior to harvest and the ensiling technique. Moreover, preservation methods, such as the addition of propionic acid to silage to prevent mould growth may influence toxin production particularly in silage that is stored for a longer period.

3. Mycotoxicosis in dairy cattle

The occurrence of clinical mycotoxicosis in cattle is a matter of controversy. While there is a common consensus that the occurrence of distinct mycotoxins, for example ergot alkaloids, can induce typical signs of intoxication, such as heat intolerance, reduced feed intake and reduced milk production in dairy herds, the impact of other mycotoxins on the health of dairy cows remains unclear. In Northern Europe, the exposure to trichothecenes occurring in grains, as well as in pasture grass is of increasing concern. Feeding experiments with deoxynivalenol, the major toxin analysed in feeds, indicated the ability of the rumen flora to degrade this toxin to DOM-1, a metabolite that lacks the epoxide moiety. DOM is considered to have a low biological activity and hence a reduced toxicity. In contrast to these experimental data, reports from Northern Europe describe a syndrome in cattle that seems to be related to the ingestion of poor grass silage, containing measurable amounts of DON. The toxic syndrome is characterised by a decrease in feed intake, reduction in the milk yield, laminitis, inflammatory reactions and fertility problems (Figure 1).

However, no experimental data are available as yet that would allow one to ascribe this syndrome to one or more individual toxins. The current hypothesis is that these symptoms are related to the exposure to multiple toxins as present in a ruminant diet.

3.1. Does the exposure to multiple toxins provide the explanation for the mycotoxicosis syndrome in dairy cows?

As indicated above, under field conditions, dairy cows can be exposed to a large diversity of mycotoxins. A critical finding is that the typical silage toxins, including patulin and mycophenolic acid exert strong antimicrobial effects. At the farm level, this effect is visible by an impairment of the rumen flora, resulting in a loss of fermentive activity of the rumen, evidenced by the appearance of non-digested fibres in the faeces. The impairment of rumen function results in subacute rumen acidosis (SARA). SARA has not only been reported following mycotoxin exposure but is a common metabolic disorder in cattle. It is well described and associated with a change of a diet

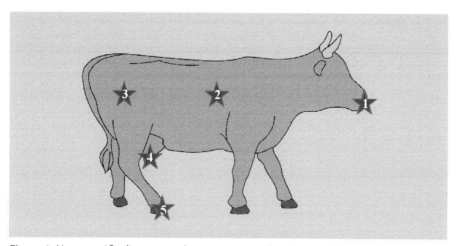

Figure 1. Non-specific disease syndrome associated with mycotoxin exposure in cattle. (1) decreased feed intake; (2) impairment of rumen function (decreased volatile fatty acids, reduced number of micro-organisms); (3) ovarian cysts, irregular heats, abortion; (4) mastitis and reduced milk yield; (5) laminitis.

and/or high concentrate intake. Affected cows experience laminitis and foot problems, their production falls below the herd average and the milk has a low fat percentage. Due to the similarity of the symptoms, it has been hypothesised that SARA may be also induced and/or accelerated by mouldy silage and the toxins produced by silage moulds.

The impaired rumen function affects also the specific barrier function of the rumen. As mentioned above, in a healthy animal the rumen flora is the first line of defence against mycotoxins in the diet. If this barrier is lost and the degrading capacity of the rumen reduced, biologically active (myco)toxins may be absorbed in the intestines. Experimental data have shown for example that a small fraction of deoxynivalenol, but also of ochratoxin A, can be found in the milk of dairy cows (Fink-Gremmels, 2008a). While these concentrations are too low to comprise a risk for human health, they serve as a clear indicator that the degrading capacity of the rumen was inappropriate. A very simple presentation of the differences between a normal cow and a cow with rumen function impairment is given in the Figure 2 to emphasis the difference.

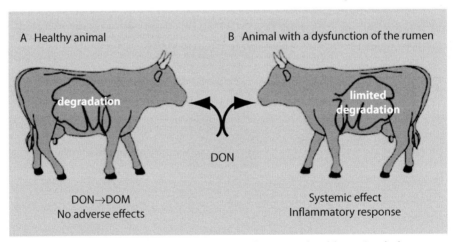

Figure 2. Two different scenarios are presented: (A) in a healthy animal, the rumen flora presents the first line of defence and degrades many mycotoxins, including DON, to biologically inactive metabolites, such as DOM. (B) In an animal with an impaired rumen function, the inactivation of DON will be incomplete, and intact DON might be absorbed from the intestines, contributing to the mycotoxicosis syndrome.

4. Mycotoxins and the immune system

A number of recent reviews have addressed the effect of mycotoxins on the immune system. The mechanisms involved are different, and comprise an impairment of the protein synthesis by many mycotoxins, including trichothecenes, but also more specific effects such as functional impairment of dendritic cells in the gastrointestinal tract and loss of epithelial integrity. One of the typical examples of a toxin that causes local adverse reactions in the gastrointestinal tract is patulin. At present these effects have been investigated only in experimental (monogastric) animals. As patulin can occurs in high amounts in silage, in might affect also the rumen wall and/or the intestines of dairy cows.

An impairment of the intestinal immune system and the induction of a generalised inflammatory response has been described in monogastric species, particularly in pigs, for other toxins as well, including deoxynivalenol and fumonisins (for review see Bouhet and Oswald, 2005). Fumonisins pass through the rumen without being degraded and deoxynivalenol might pass through the rumen if silage moulds impair its flora. Hence, comparable effects on the immune system in cattle can not be excluded.

Of special interest is the putative role of *Aspergillus fumigatus* in the pathogenesis of mycotoxicoses in cattle. While this *Aspergillus* species is considered to be part of the normal rumen flora, its occurrence in intestines has been associated with a severe disease syndrome (inflammatory and haemorrhagic bowel disease). *Aspergillus fumigatus* produces in animal (and human) tissues the mycotoxin gliotoxin, which is among the most potent immunosuppressive agents identified in nature.

5. Targets of intervention

Under current agricultural practice, the occurrence of many *Fusarium* toxins, *Neothyphodium* toxins and aflatoxins are considered to be unavoidable in feed materials. In turn, current efforts focus not only on measures that might reduce the rate of contamination of food and feed commodities, but are aiming to identify strategies that mitigate or reduce the adverse effects of mycotoxins in the animal. In dairy cows and cattle, these intervention strategies should be directed towards:
- Improvement of the rumen flora using live yeast or other pre- and probiotics that are known rumen flora stimulants.

- Reduction of exposure to mycotoxins through the use of compounds, such as aluminium silicates (>40 different compounds) and yeast-derived polymeric glucomannans that reduce the absorption of, and consequent exposure to mycotoxins.
- Support of the innate immune system with antioxidants and/or selenium that can alleviate oxidative stress, as well as the direct immuno-suppressive effects of individual mycotoxins.

6. Conclusions

Adverse effects of individual mycotoxins, such as ergot alkaloids, have been intensively investigated in ruminants. This applies also to the group of aflatoxins, as one of the metabolites, aflatoxin M_1 can be excreted with milk and its occurrence in milk is monitored within the frame of food safety objectives. However, the current knowledge on the possible adverse effects of other mycotoxins, commonly found in feed materials on ruminants, is very limited. The lack of data is explained by the general assumption that the rumen microbiological flora is able to degrade and inactivate all mycotoxins. However, accumulating evidence suggests that this paradigm needs to be amended, as animals are generally exposed to a complex mixture of mycotoxins, originating from different sources. In addition, in the presence of other metabolic disorders, such as SARA, animals might be more sensitive to mycotoxins. Further investigations should aim to provide a closer insight in the effects of mycotoxins in the annual cycle of a dairy cow (Fink-Gremmels, 2008b).

References

Bouhet, S. and I.P.Oswald, 2005. The effect of mycotoxins, fungal food contaminants, on the intestinal epithelial cell-derived innate immune response. Veterinary Immunology and Immunopathology **108**:199-209.

Fink-Gremmels, J., 2005. Mycotoxins in forages. In:Diaz, D.E. (Ed). The mycotoxin blue book. Nottingham University Press, Nottingham, United Kingdom, pp 249-268.

Fink-Gremmels, J., 2008a. Mycotoxins in cattle feeds and carry-over to dairy milk: a review. *Food Additives and Contaminants* **25**: 172-180.

Fink-Gremmels, J., 2008b. The role of mycotoxins in the health and performance of dairy cows. *Veterinary Journal* **176**:84-92.

Jouany, J. and D. Diaz, 2005. Effects of mycotoxins in ruminants. In: Diaz, D.E. (Ed.). The mycotoxin blue book. Nottingham University Press, Nottingham, United Kingdom, pp 295-321.

Mansfield, M.A., A.D. Jones and G.A. Kuldau, 2008. Contamination of fresh and ensiled maize by multiple *Penicillium* mycotoxins. *Phytopathology* **98**:330-336.

Schardl, J., H. Jensen and J. Latge, 1996. *Epichloe festucae* and related mutualistic symbionts of grasses. *Fungal Genetics and Biology* **33**:69-82.

Keyword index

A

acidosis 34, 38, 48, 65, 66, 75
  – subacute rumen (SARA) 49-53, 64-66, 87, 88, 90
advisor 11, 18-20, 22
aflatoxins 83, 85, 89, 90
alpha-tocopherol 26
antioxidant 71, 74, 75, 90
Aspergillus 86, 89

B

behaviour 13, 14, 16, 18, 20, 22, 52, 53, 66
beta-carotene 26
biotin 71, 72
body
  – condition 11, 50
  – weight 29

C

calcium 25, 34, 45, 46, 48, 49, 53, 73, 74
calf health 25, 27, 28
cattle health 11, 12, 16, 20-22
chlorine 49
claw 61-63, 65-67, 69, 71, 72, 75, 76
cobalt 74
colostrum 25-29
communication 13, 16, 19-22
copper 25, 74

D

deoxynivalenol 84, 86, 88, 89
dietary
  – fibre 51
  – protein 67, 68
Dietary Cation Anion Difference 48
digital

  – cushion 63, 64, 71, 74
  – dermatitis 61
direct feed microbials 52
displaced abomasum 34, 42, 47, 52, 53
dry cow 25, 26, 35, 40, 41, 48, 49, 51, 53
Dutch udder health
  – centre 23
  – program 14

E

education 11, 18
endometritis 34
ergot alkaloids 84-86, 90

F

failure of passive transfer 28
fatty liver 35-39, 41, 42, 53
feed intake 33, 38, 39, 41, 43, 44, 47, 50-53, 86, 87
fertility 12, 33, 35, 40, 42, 46, 53, 87
fumonisins 83-85, 89
Fusarium 84, 89

G

gliotoxin 89
glucomannans 90

H

horn capsule 62-64, 66
hypocalcaemia 34, 35, 44-47, 49, 53

I

immunity 27, 29, 42, 47, 83, 84
immunosuppression 34, 35, 39, 42, 45, 46, 50
iodine 26
iron 25

Printed in the United States
by Baker & Taylor Publisher Services